EMERGENCY
& Disaster Preparedness
for Health Professionals

Second Edition

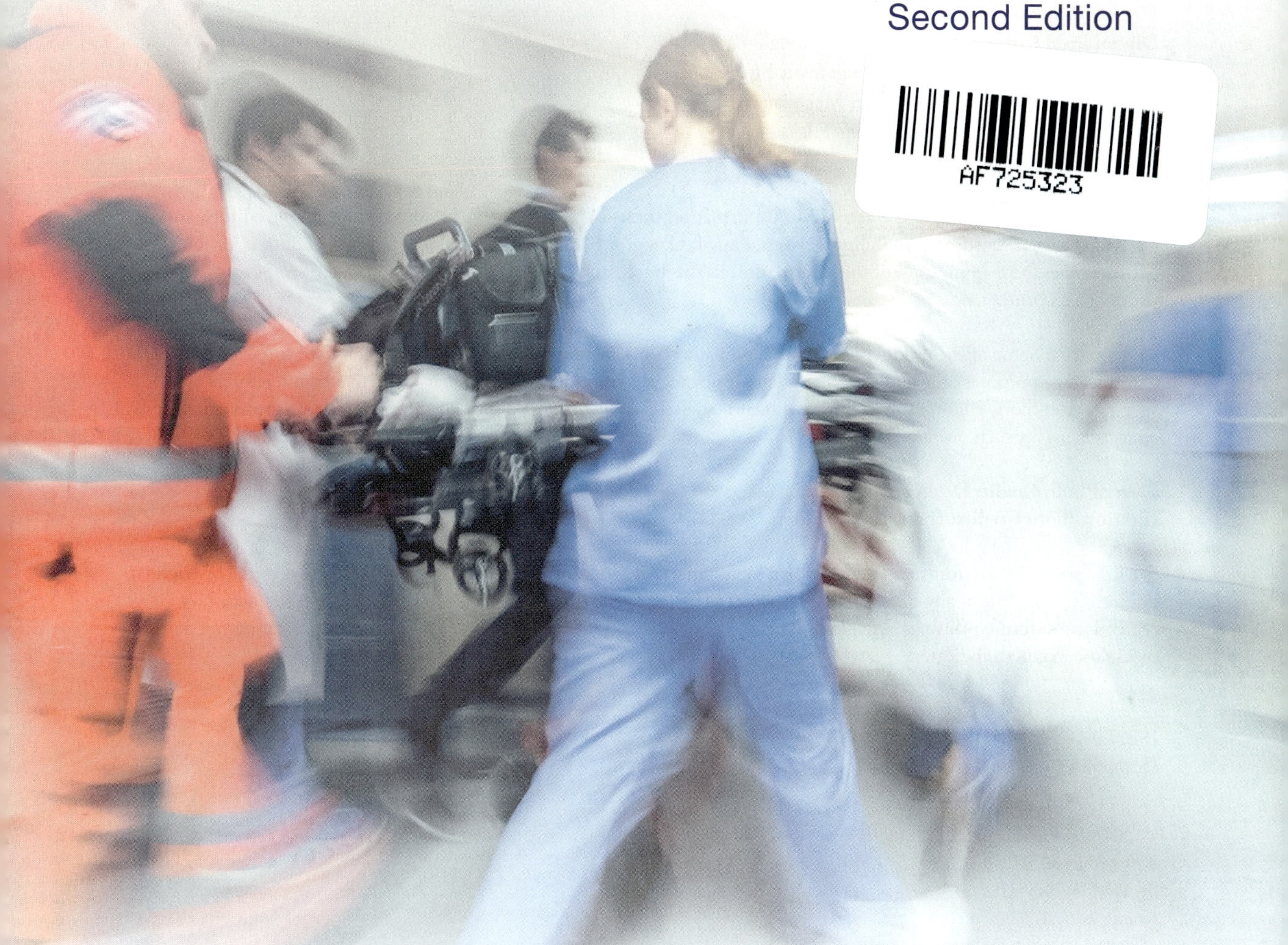

Linda Young Landesman, DrPH, MSW

PARADIGM
EDUCATION SOLUTIONS

St. Paul

Division President: Linda Hein
Vice President, Content Management: Christine Hurney
Managing Editor: Carley Fruzzetti
Developmental Editor: Marybeth Lorbiecki
Director of Production: Timothy W. Larson
Production Editor: Jen Weaverling
Cover and Text Designer and Senior Design and Production Specialist: Valerie King
Senior Design and Production Specialist: Jack Ross
Copy Editor: Audrey Suzanne Clinton
Proofreader: Margaret P. Roeske
Indexer: Terry Casey
Vice President, Digital Solutions: Chuck Bratton
Digital Projects Manager: Tom Modl
Digital Solutions Manager: Gerry Yumul
Digital Production Manager: Aaron Esnough
Vice President, Sales and Marketing: Scott Burns
Director of Marketing: Lara Weber McLellan
Product Marketing Manager: Selena Hicks

Cover Photo Credit: © vo/gettyimages.com
Interior Photo Credits: Following the index.

ISBN 978-0-76388-142-9 (print)
ISBN 978-0-76388-140-5 (digital)

875 Montreal Way
St. Paul, MN 55102
Email: educate@emcp.com
Website: ParadigmEducation.com

Printed in the United States of America

26 25 24 23 22 21 20 19 18 17 1 2 3 4 5 6 7 8 9 10

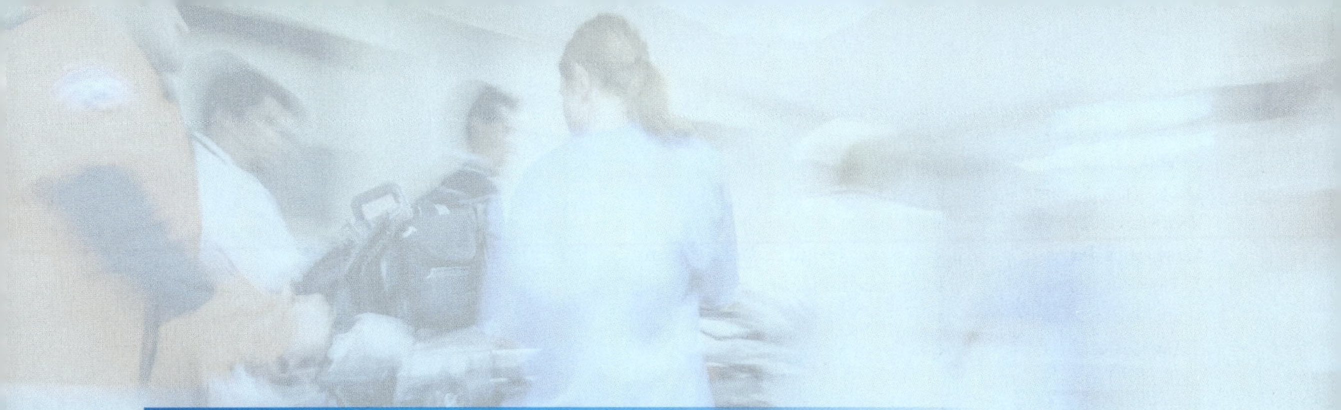

Brief Contents

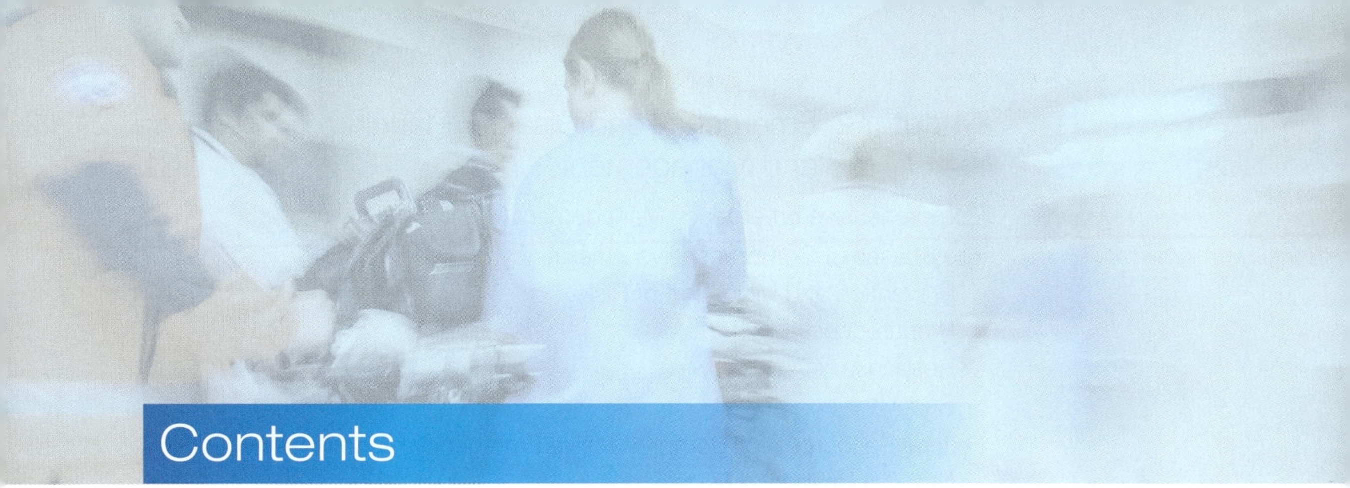

Contents

Preface

Recent disasters, such as hurricanes, mass shootings and other acts of terrorism, and and infectious disease outbreaks, have emphasized why emergency preparedness is a local and national priority. Healthcare systems must ready themselves and their staff to respond effectively to these kinds of emergencies and disasters. Allied health professionals play very important roles.

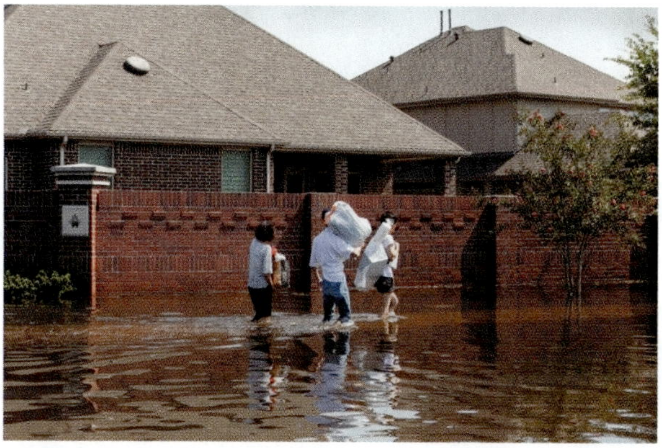

Residents walk in flood waters in a Houston suburb in the aftermath of Hurricane Harvey.

When you become a health professional, how will you contribute to effective emergency response? What do you need to know?

The second edition of *Emergency & Disaster Preparedness for Health Professionals* distills the essential, up-to-date information regarding how communities, healthcare facilities, and health professionals prepare and respond in these events.

Written by the premiere public health specialist in the field, this pioneering book will teach you the fundamentals of emergency and disaster response and how to apply your skills in this challenging context. With this knowledge, you will be prepared to meet your professional responsibilities to your employer, your patients, and your community.

Program Features and Resources

Use this text to explore key concepts, agencies, organizations, processes, and terms related to emergency and disaster preparedness and response. Learn about the four phases of comprehensive emergency management and see how the phases are applied in real-world case studies: Hurricane Katrina, the Boston Marathon bombings, and Ebola Virus Disease.

The following features provide engaging content for faster, deeper learning:

- A list of learning objectives at the beginning of each chapter that focuses on what you need to know
- A *Key Acronyms* box at the beginning of each chapter that provides the terms, agencies, and procedures commonly referred to by their acronyms
- *Key Terms* that are set in bold, defined in the text or in boxes, listed at the end of each chapter, and provided in the glossary
- Margin tips that highlight key concepts and additional information
- *A Closer Look* and *Heroes Corner* boxes that add concrete examples or describe concepts in more detail
- Web icons appear on footers to indicate pages that have informational web links and clickable links in the eBook pull-down menus.
- A chapter summary, review questions, and higher-level research and dialog questions end each chapter to help you integrate and assess your understanding

eBook

Emergency & Disaster Preparedness for Health Professionals, Second Edition, also comes to you in an electronic format. The web-based, password-protected eBook features dynamic navigation tools, including bookmarking, a linked table of contents, and access to additional study tools. These include:

- Glossary and flash cards
- Supplements, such as "Social Media Tools"
- Website resource list and sources reference list

NEW! eChapter Add-Ons Available

Profession-specific eChapters provide additional hands-on laboratory activities and projects. See **http://EmDPrep2.ParadigmEducation.com/CourseOfferings** for a list of available eChapters, such as "Pharmacy and Preparedness."

Instructor eResources

The instructor resources that accompany this textbook are located on the *Instructor eResources*, a password-protected eBook that is only available to instructors. These resources include course-planning documents, chapter lessons, PowerPoint presentations, and optional hands-on labs.

About the Author

Dr. Linda Young Landesman, DrPH, MSW, BA, is a nationally recognized expert in emergency preparedness who has a long and distinguished career in public health working as a clinician, administrator, educator, policymaker, and author. She is considered one of the key pioneers in the field of public health preparedness. Dr. Landesman was the Principal Investigator for the first national curriculum on the public health management of disasters, developed through a cooperative agreement with the Association of Schools of Public Health and sponsored by the Centers for Disease Control and Prevention. She also developed national standards for Emergency Medical Services response. Dr. Landesman is currently on the faculty of the Public Health Practice Program at the University of Massachusetts–Amherst, where she teaches research methods and public health emergency management online.

Dr. Landesman retired in 2012 after 16 years as Assistant Vice President, Office of Professional Services and Affiliations, at the New York City Health and Hospitals Corporation (HHC). Appointments to numerous committees and community boards have included among others: the Regional Advisory Committee for the New York State Commission on Health Care Facilities for the Twenty-First Century; Commissioners' Advisory Committee, New York City Department of Health and Mental Hygiene; Advisory Committee, World Trade Center (WTC) Evacuation Study; Weapons of Mass Destruction Advisory Council, New York City Department of Health; Emergency Preparedness Council, New York City Health and Hospitals Corporation; Center for Public Health Preparedness, Mailman School of Public Health of Columbia University; F30 accelerated writing groups and content expert, ASTM International; and the Disabled in Disaster Advisory Group, Orange County, CA.

Dr. Landesman has been a member of the American Public Health Association, Public Health Association of New York City, the New York State Public Health Association, Hermann Biggs Society, and a Fellow at the New York Academy of Medicine. She has edited or authored 10 books, including the landmark book, *Landesman's Public Health Management of Disasters: The Practice Guide*, now in its fourth edition. This book is the go-to book for everyone in the field. She has also written dozens of journal articles and book chapters. Dr. Landesman earned her BA and MSW degrees from the University of Michigan. She received her DrPH in health policy and management from the Columbia University Mailman School of Public Health. Her doctoral dissertation focused on hospital preparedness for chemical accidents and won the Doctoral Dissertation Award from the Health Services Improvement Fund in 1990.

Acknowledgments

The quality of this book is a testament to the many contributors and reviewers who participated in the creation of *Emergency and Disaster Preparedness*, Second Edition. We offer a heartfelt thank-you for your commitment to producing high-quality instructional materials for allied health students.

Reviewers and Contributors

Scott Becker, MS
Executive Director
Association of Public Health Laboratories

Noah Brown
Senior Public Affairs & Media Relations Officer
Massachusetts General Hospital

Julie Burger, MPH, CPH, CHES, CPhT
Pharmacy Technician Program Director
Pensacola State College

Chief Master Sergeant Jason Burger
United States Air Force

Constance Talcott Johnston Doyle, MD
Michigan-1 Disaster Medical Assistance Team (DMAT)

Karen M. Daughtery, CPhT, ASCT
Program Chair, Pharmacy Technology
Vincennes University

Kimberly S Glassman, PhD, RN, NEA-BC, FAAN
Senior Vice President, Patient Care Services and Chief Nursing Officer
NYU Langone Medical Center

Gabriela Grygus, MBA, RHIA
Senior Director, Health Information Management
NYU Langone Health System

John B. Herman, MD
Associate Chief, Department of Psychiatry
Massachusetts General Hospital

Pamela Holmes
Director of Consumer and Regulatory Affairs, Ultratec, Inc.

Barbara Ilardi, MPA, CDN, CPH
Public Information Officer
Putnam County Department of Health

June Kailes
Disability Policy Consultant

Grace Kubin, PhD
Director
Texas Department of State Health Services Laboratory

Chris N. Mangal, MPH
Director, Public Health Preparedness and Response
Association of Public Health Laboratories

Linda McCormick
Executive Assistant
Massachusetts General Hospital

Elina Pierce, MSP, CPhT
Chair, Pharmacy Technician Program
Southeast Community College

Hiran Ratnayake
Manager of Media and Government Relations
Christiana Care Health System

Laura Sheiman, MD
Assistant Professor, Department of Radiology and Biomedical Imaging
Yale School of Medicine

Nyle L. Salley, MPH, EMT-B
Program Specialist (EMS Division)
Westchester County Dept. of Emergency Services

Lauren Ann Witbart, MEd, EdS, MPH
Centers for Disease Control and Prevention
Office of Public Health Preparedness and Response

Irina Zusman
Director of Coding & Clinical Data Improvement Initiatives
NYU Langone Medical Center

Advisory Board Members

Paradigm Education Solutions would also like to thank our Advisory Board members for contributing to the development of this book.

Irene Banuelos-Villatoro, BS, CPhT, RPhT
San Jacinto College North

Nicole Barriera, CPhT
Pikes Peak Community College

Hertencia Bowe, MS
Fisher College

Mark Bruton, MED, CPhT
Education and Pharmacy Consultant

Christine Bushaw, MEd, RHIT
Rochester Community and Technical College

Lynette Hessling, MSHI, RHIA, CHTS-PW, CHTS-TR
Ultimate Medical Academy

Kevin Hope, RPh
Clinical Pharmacy Education Specialist, freeCE

Jorell Lawrence, MSA, CPC
Trinity Health, Central Michigan University

Anne LaVance, CPhT
Delgado Community College

Wendy Almeda Lubin BS, CPhT
Front Range Community College

Telma O'Neal, MEd, BS
Virginia College

Sandra Rains, MPA, MBA, RHIA
Nationwide Children's Hospital

Terri Randolph, MBA/HCM, CAHI, CBCS, CEHRS
McKesson, University of Phoenix

Nader Rassaei, MD, MA, BS, CPhT
El Paso Community College

Andrea Redman, Pharm D, BCPS
Emory Healthcare

Marcia Sharp, EdD, RHIA
University of Tennessee

Hannah Brooke Stokely, BS, CPhT
Southeastern Institute, Pfeiffer Institute

Veronica Velasquez BA, PhTR, CPhT
Austin Community College

Wanda Ziemba, EJD, MFA, RHIA, CCS, CHC, CHCO/CHCC, CPC
City College of San Francisco

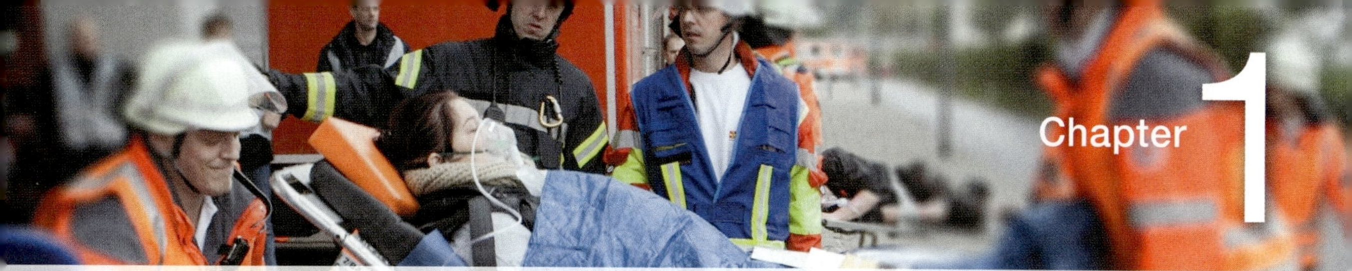

Chapter 1

Emergencies, Disasters, and Health Care

What You Will Learn

- Basic terms used in emergency and disaster preparedness
- Reasons for an all-hazards approach to preparing for emergencies and disasters
- Various types of natural disasters (both seasonal and geological) and human-caused disasters, and their direct and indirect impacts
- The dangers of infectious diseases that can become epidemics or pandemics
- The threat of emerging infectious diseases and bioterrorism
- The roles of healthcare coalitions, facilities, and personnel

Imagine that an emergency or disaster strikes your community today. You are a health professional working in a hospital, long-term care facility, medical office, or pharmacy. What should you expect? Will you know what to do?

This book will prepare you to carry out your duties as a health professional during such an event. You will learn how to prepare and respond effectively, safely, and confidently. This chapter provides a basic orientation to common emergencies and disasters.

An Emergency and Disaster Orientation

What is an emergency? How are emergencies and disasters similar and how are they different? What do employers and communities expect health professionals to know about emergency and disaster response? Let's start with the basics.

Basic Terms

Emergencies are situations that threaten public safety, health, and welfare. Some emergencies are limited, such as a house fire or a shooting. Others are larger in scope and require a greater response, such as a hurricane. Hospital staff use the term *emergency* to mean any situation in which a patient requires immediate care or a higher level of care. However, the field of public health defines an **emergency** as a broader event involving groups of people. **Emergency response** is a coordinated local action by the town, city, metropolitan area, or county. The local response involves the police, fire department, Emergency Medical Services (EMS), and healthcare facilities.

An emergency that requires outside assistance from the federal government is defined as a **disaster**. The disaster assistance provided often includes healthcare professionals, medications, and medical equipment and supplies.

An emergency or disaster event is known as an **incident**. An incident can be as specific as a mass shooting or a bombing in a single area or as widespread as a hurricane with many response sites.

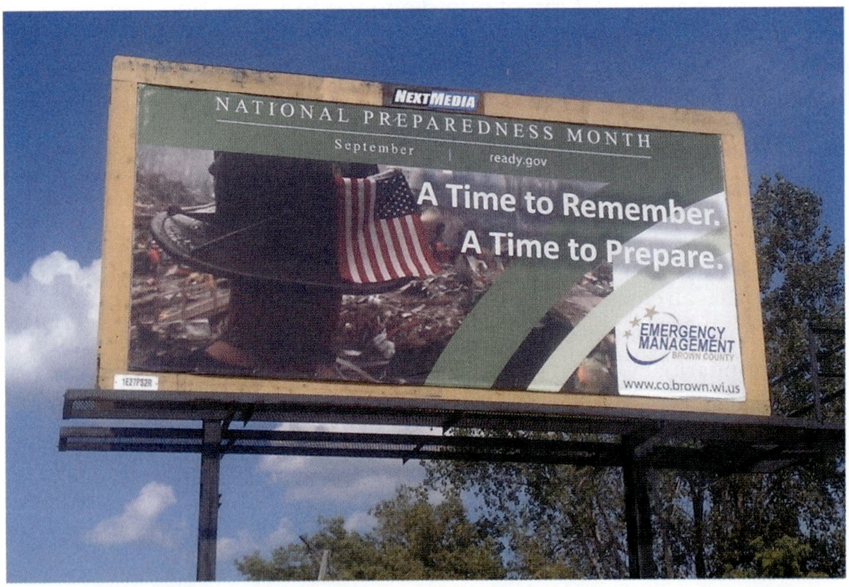
NEXTMEDIA
NATIONAL PREPAREDNESS MONTH
September
ready.gov
A Time to Remember.
A Time to Prepare.
EMERGENCY MANAGEMENT
www.co.brown.wi.us

This billboard in Green Bay, Wisconsin, reminds people about the importance of preparing for emergency and disasters.

Key Acronyms	
CBRNE	chemical, biological, radiological, nuclear, and high-yield explosives
CDC	Centers for Disease Control and Prevention
EMS	Emergency Medical Service
EMTs	emergency medical technicians
FEMA	Federal Emergency Management Agency
HCCs	healthcare coalitions
NGOs	nongovernmental organizations
NOAA	National Oceanic and Atmospheric Administration
SARS	severe acute respiratory syndrome
USGS	US Geological Survey

First responders are the initial professionals to arrive at the scene and may be emergency medical technicians (EMTs) or paramedics, firefighters, and/or the police. Additional responders may include members of the healthcare system, National Guard, civic groups, volunteer organizations, and search and rescue teams. Specific action plans for response will be employed at every individual incident site. **Victims** are the people who are impacted, injured, or become ill as a result of an emergency or disaster. **NGOs**, as they are commonly known, are **nongovernmental organizations**. Many NGOs from the community, region, nation, and even other nations get involved in disaster response, including the American Red Cross and religiously affiliated groups.

Several other terms are commonly used. **Emergency and disaster preparedness** is the act of making plans to prevent, respond to, and recover from these devastating events. Government agencies, healthcare systems, community groups, and even families take part in preparedness.

Though emergencies and disasters vary in size and scope, they present many similar challenges. For example, warning people, evacuating them, and providing shelter can be handled in similar ways in most disasters. Because of these similarities, the recommended approach is called **all-hazards planning**. All-hazards planning provides general preparation and training that can be applied in a wide range of emergency situations. This approach is more effective and practical than training for every potential type of emergency.

Health professionals clearly play key roles in any emergency response. They bring specialized clinical and administrative skills, and they understand how healthcare systems work. They are skilled at providing care to people who are injured, ill, or worried. Becoming ready to handle a disaster requires preparation and training.

Expand Your Knowledge

Emergency Medical Service (EMS) is the community-oriented system for providing emergency treatment and transportation to hospitals.

After Hurricane Katrina devastated neighborhoods with flooding, this patient was evacuated by a medevac helicopter. Approximately 1,800 people died as a result of the hurricane, but many more were saved by the emergency and disaster response teams.

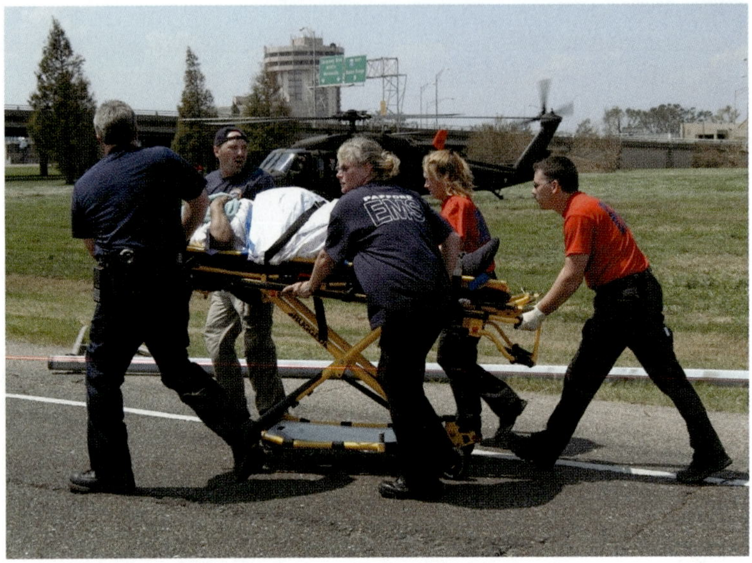

The Impacts of Natural Disasters

To know how to properly respond in a disaster, it is essential to understand the many ways that different types of disasters can affect the health of a community. Some ways are obvious, but others are not. For instance, if many people arrive at a hospital's emergency room at the same time, the facility is likely to have insufficient staffing to provide adequate care or all the required medicines and supplies.

In an earthquake, we expect that people will be injured by falling debris, and in wildfires, people will be harmed by smoke, ash, and burns if they can not evacuate in time. These are direct impacts. But disasters also have indirect impacts that are not specific to each type of crisis. Consider that when homes are destroyed, people lose their medications, walkers, canes, and even their glasses. This section explores some of the direct and indirect impacts of disasters that result from natural causes. The next section will examine the impacts of disasters that are the result of human actions or activities. The final section will discuss infectious diseases to which few people have immunity.

Natural disasters are caused by meteorological events of extreme or unexpected weather, or by geological events. Natural disasters include floods, hurricanes, tornadoes, mudslides and landslides, heat waves, wildfires, blizzards and ice storms, avalanches, earthquakes, tsunamis, and volcanic eruptions. Clearly, these disasters vary widely in the severity and types of damage they cause. You need to be prepared to meet the challenges associated with the disasters most likely to occur in your area.

The first group of disasters to follow are those caused by severe or extended weather conditions. In the US, the **National Oceanic and Atmospheric Administration (NOAA)** tracks weather systems and alerts communities when a potentially dangerous weather event may soon occur.

The second group of disasters result from geological changes in the earth. The **US Geological Survey (USGS)** is the agency that helps monitor and alert communities about potential geological disasters. It provides science about the natural hazards that threaten lives and livelihoods, and the health of our ecosystems and environment. The USGS also studies the scenarios that can cause problems and the impacts of climate and land-use change.

Expand Your Knowledge

For NOAA weather watch and alerts, go to its webpage at **www.noaa.gov/weather**.

For real-time or near real-time information and data on current geological conditions, such as earthquakes and volcanoes, and earth observations, go to **www.usgs.gov**.

Floods

Floods occur more frequently than any other type of disaster. They happen when huge amounts of rain fall, generally over several days, causing a river or stream to overflow into the surrounding areas. Flooding can also occur from a rapid melting of snow upstream. Citizens usually feel they can trust the standing infrastructures to hold back the waters and stop any floods from becoming overwhelming and dangerous. However, excessive rainfall or snow melting may cause levees or dams to break, releasing huge amounts of water in a short time.

People who live in areas that flood regularly try to be prepared for seasonal overflows, but they may not be ready for huge amounts of water. Breaks in

Expand Your Knowledge

In February 2017, about 188,000 residents were ordered to evacuate near the Oroville Dam in Northern California. Rising rainwater put pressure on the dam, and a side channel crumbled. Massive amounts of water rushed out, endangering the area.

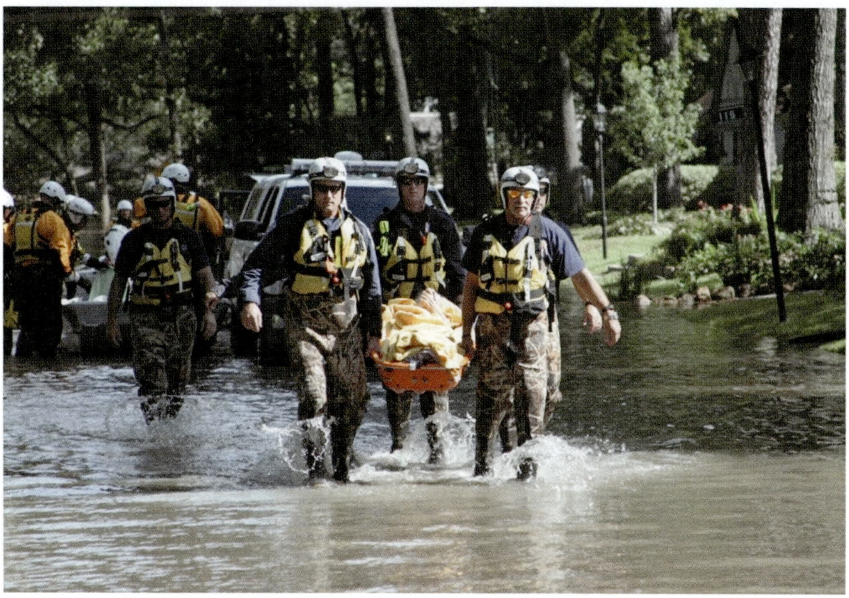

FEMA's Urban Search and Rescue Teams from Nebraska Task Force 1 remove a victim from a neighborhood impacted by flooding from Hurricane Harvey.

Be Aware

Manhole covers often pop out of place in floods. People have died during floods when they walked through waist deep water and fell through manhole openings into the flooded sewer system.

Be Aware

Standing water from floods or hurricanes can become breeding grounds for mosquitoes that may carry infectious diseases.

infrastructures can cause **flash flooding**, or sudden fast-moving water. Most flood-related deaths occur from flash flooding. People commonly die when they try to drive, wade, or ride bicycles through water that is flowing very rapidly, not realizing how deep or how powerful the current is.

Floods can affect the health of people in the community in many other ways too. Sewage systems may overflow into the floodwaters. People then develop gastrointestinal and skin diseases from exposure to contaminated water. If the electrical power goes out, refrigerated and frozen food spoil, and refrigerated medications lose their effectiveness. Patients with chronic health conditions often develop complications because they cannot access their medications or usual medical care.

After flood-waters subside, life does not quickly go back to normal. Cleanup takes a long time, and many structures and cars cannot be saved because of the damage. Mold grows quickly and causes illnesses or exacerbates existing health conditions, particularly respiratory diseases.

Hurricanes

Besides coming from inland storms, flooding can accompany hurricanes. These powerful storms travel in from the oceans, bringing heavy rain and swirling, intense winds that cover a wide region. The high-velocity winds (from 74 mph to over 157 mph) move in large circular patterns around a quiet center called the eye. The eye can be 20 to 40 miles in width.

Be Aware

When Hurricane Harvey hit in August of 2017, it broke rain records for a storm in the continental US with over 51 inches (17 feet) of rain in some areas of Texas. This record rainfall caused flooding in areas well beyond normal flood zones.

As the storm moves at a rate between 10 and 20 miles per hour, the initial hurricane winds will tear through an area, and then there will be a quiet period as the eye passes over. It may seem as if the storm is over, but then the winds will howl again when the other side of the hurricane hits. The enormous amount of rain often causes flooding when water pours over riverbanks or tidal areas or breaks through levees. Neighboring communities may not be able to help each other when they are also affected.

Most hurricanes on the Atlantic coast hit shore from August through October. Meteorologists can usually predict, with reasonable accuracy, the timing and location of the storm striking land. Their predictions make it possible to warn communities and advise them to activate disaster plans.

Despite having advance weather warnings, however, residents do not always follow the safety or evacuation guidelines to prevent injuries and keep their food and water safe. People can drown or be injured by electrical wires that have fallen. They can be cut from flying debris or suffer fractures due to falling trees and flying objects. They may be isolated without water or food that is safe to drink and eat.

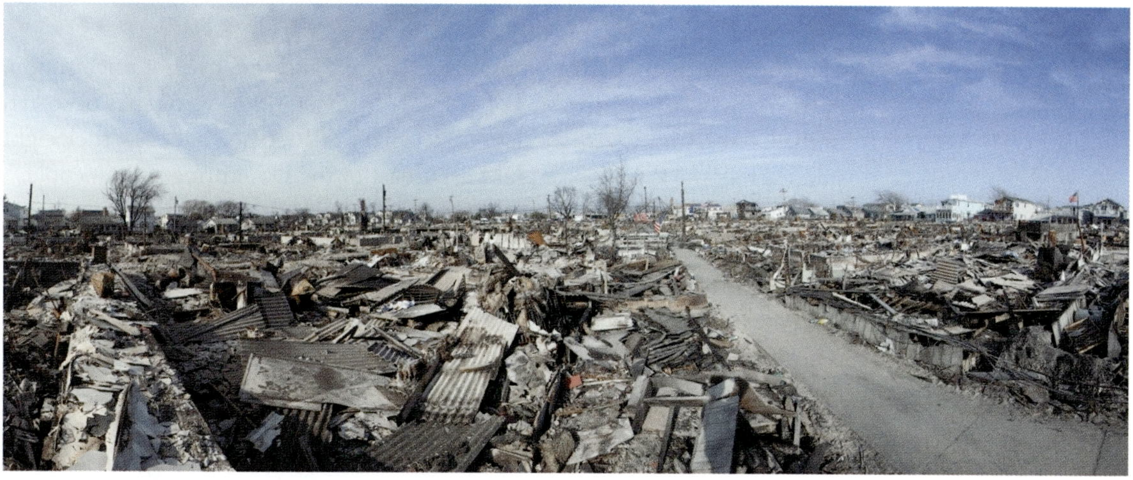

Hurricanes strike the coastlines of the Gulf of Mexico and Atlantic Ocean nearly every year. Strong winds, heavy rains, and flooding destroy the buildings and endanger life. These are some of the houses destroyed by Hurricane Sandy on November 12, 2012, in the Breezy Point neighborhood of Queens in New York.

A Closer Look

Hospitals Facing Floods

Hurricane Sandy was so severe that it destroyed homes and caused flooding over 900 miles—a much larger area than is typical with hurricanes. Almost 120 people died during and after the storm. Most people died from drowning; many died because they did not evacuate.

When long-term care facilities or hospitals must be swiftly evacuated, managing the move can be very difficult. For example, two medical centers along the East River in New York City faced these challenges during Hurricane Sandy in 2012.

At New York University Langone Medical Center, additional staff were called in to help discharge patients, and hospital staff had to locate available beds in other hospitals for those too sick to go home. With the power out from flooding, patients had to be carried down the stairs. Evacuation was particularly complicated with intensive-care premature babies and others on life-support equipment. But the staff got the patients out safely.

For a dramatic recounting of how Bellevue Hospital Center (now NYC Health+ Hospitals Bellevue) handled the storm, go to: **http://EmDPrp2.ParadigmEducation.com/bellevue-hurricane**.

Expand Your Knowledge

To learn more about hurricanes and Hurricane Sandy, watch this National Geographic video: **http://EmDPrp2.ParadigmEducation.com/hurricanes-101**.

Tornadoes

Tornadoes are one of nature's most severe storms, and they are not uncommon, particularly in the Midwest. For instance, almost 1,000 tornadoes occurred in the US in 2016. Over two days in February 2016, 61 tornadoes struck eight states across the Gulf Coast and East Coast of the US, killing seven people.

Tornadoes usually develop during severe thunderstorms when winds from different directions collide in the sky and begin to twirl around each other. The winds form funnel shapes as they rotate. Winds in some funnels have been measured at speeds of more than 300 miles per hour, causing death and destruction when the funnels touch down. A tornado's on-the-ground path is usually between 300 and 500 yards across but can be as wide as a mile. While touching ground, it can destroy all structures in its way. Tornadoes have traveled across the land as far as 50 miles, but the average distance is 26 miles per tornado. A particularly tumultuous storm can spawn numerous tornadoes.

Many communities use siren systems to warn people that a tornado has been sighted, so that they can take shelter. Although tornadoes can occur in all the lower 48 states, they occur most often in the South and Midwest.

Expand Your Knowledge

To learn more about tornadoes, watch this National Geographic video: http://EmDPrp2.ParadigmEducation.com/tornadoes-101.

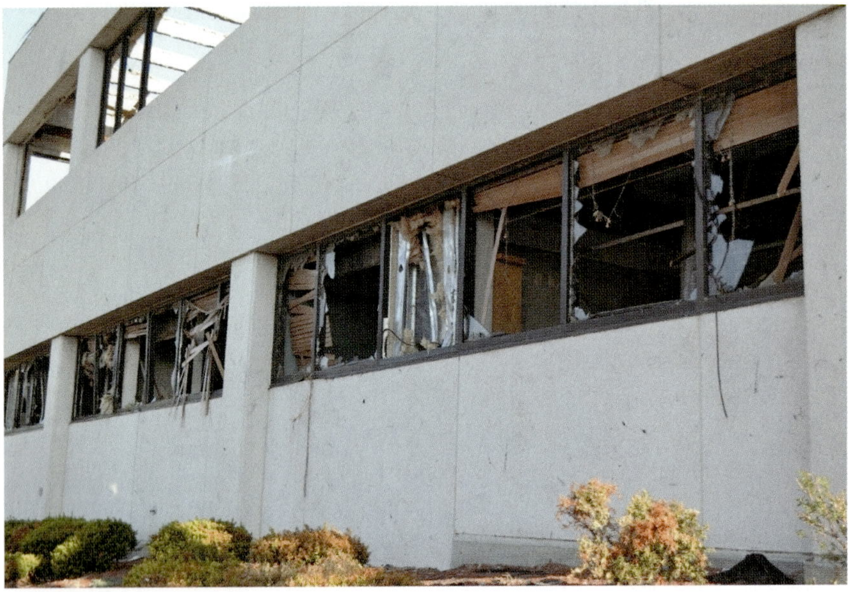

On Sunday afternoon, May 22, 2011, a tornado flattened buildings in Joplin, Missouri. It was a mile wide in places, with multiple funnels. Though sirens sounded 20 minutes in advance, many people did not hear them. The tornado killed 158 people and injured more than 1,100. The healthcare system was crippled when the Greenbriar Nursing Home was leveled and the St. John's Regional Medical Center was destroyed, as shown here.

The Midwest and Southeast must be aware particularly during the months of March through May. Healthcare facilities must be especially ready during these months in tornado-prone regions.

People can be crushed or injured from collapsing structures and flying debris or from being knocked over or picked up by the high winds. The stress of tornadoes can cause some people to have heart attacks. Power lines are often knocked down. While the electricity is out, people with chronic illnesses may have their medications go bad, or their medical equipment may not work. People can also become ill from consuming unsafe water or food.

Mudslides and Landslides

After storms and heavy rains, especially those that cause floods, mudslides may occur. In a mudslide, tons of rock, earth, or debris mixed with water pour down a hill or mountain, burying things in their path. Landslides are similar but do not contain water. The areas most at risk for landslides and mudslides are wherever wildfires or logging have occurred, or where construction has changed the shape of hills.

Droughts, earthquakes, and volcanic eruptions can cause slides. When roadways are covered by the debris from slides, traffic accidents and backups may occur, and people may not be able to get to health facilities for care.

Expand Your Knowledge

On March 22, 2014, with no immediate warning, a mountainside collapsed onto 49 homes near Oso, Washington, northwest of Seattle. The slide killed 43 people and buried parts of State Highway 530. To view landslides in action, see: **http://EmDPrp2.ParadigmEducation.com/Oso-landslides**.

Heat Waves

When the daytime temperature stays high for several days in a row and does not drop at night, this is considered a heat wave. Older adults, infants, and people who are obese may have difficulty adjusting to the heat. This can lead to health problems, which are often exacerbated when both the temperature and the humidity are high. More people are affected by heat waves in June and July in the US, as compared to other months, because it is easier to adapt to the heat as summer goes on.

People usually do not get sick at the start of a heat wave. The body can initially adjust to the heat through perspiration and varying blood circulation. However, when the body cannot cool itself adequately because of exposure to extended heat, the body temperature rises dangerously. This can lead to illness and death. The elderly are most prone to dying from heat waves. Medical facilities can expect more patients during these times of intense, prolonged heat.

Wildfires

Heat waves can lead to low moisture levels and high fire risks, especially in areas that have been experiencing low rainfall for extended periods of drought. Wildfires can be ignited by lightning strikes or a spark from the rails as a train passes. They can also be started by arson or people who are careless. More

Annually, an average of more than 7 million acres are burned by more than 73,000 wildfires in the US. Structures and communities in the path of a wildfire must be evacuated. Regional healthcare facilities need to be ready to handle the widespread respiratory problems.

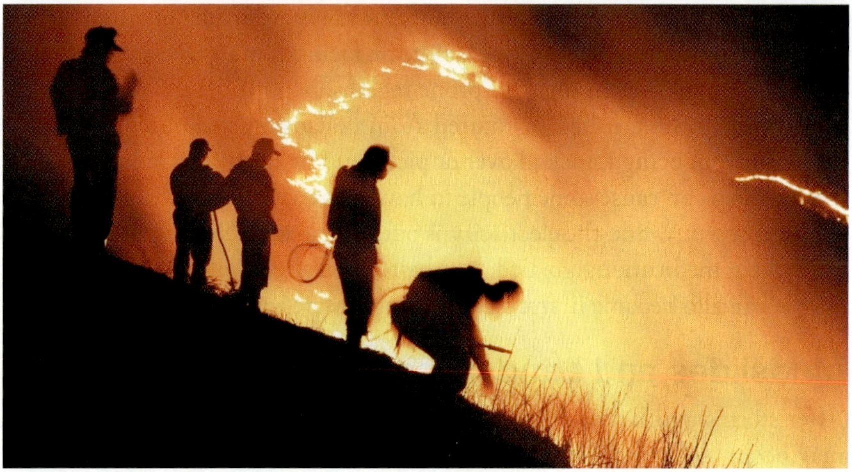

than four out of five wildfires are started by discarded cigarettes or campfires not carefully extinguished.

Wildfires spread quickly in forests or natural areas if there are windy, dry weather conditions. The flames, heat, smoke, and ash cause burns and inhalation injuries, and exacerbate respiratory conditions. If toxic substances or building materials catch fire, they may release poisonous gases. Wildfires can also trigger stress-related cardiovascular events while people are fighting or fleeing the fire.

The number of wildfires has increased since the 1980s in the US. For instance, in the late fall of 2016, the Southeast had little rain and the humidity was very low. Over 50 major wildfires burned an excess of 119,000 acres in eight states. More than 6,300 firefighters fought these fires, some coming from as far as the state of Washington. Although no lives were lost, some people suffered minor injuries, and hundreds of people went to emergency rooms and doctor's offices with respiratory problems due to the unhealthy air and smoke. The helicopter used for medical rescue at the University of Tennessee Medical Center did not fly for a week because of concerns about exposing patients and the pilots to dangerous respiratory conditions. The smoke also affected animals.

Blizzards and Ice Storms

In contrast to the summer heat waves and wildfires, winter blizzards and ice storms bring intense cold temperatures and low wind chills, huge accumulations of snow, shifting snowdrifts, sleet and black ice, high winds, and blinding snow. Flying, driving, and walking are hazardous in these conditions. In such storms, it is difficult to get emergency vehicles to those who are injured on the roadway or for hospital staff to reach the healthcare facilities for their shifts. The National Weather Service usually predicts winter storms in advance and provides warnings so that communities can prepare.

Most deaths during winter storms occur in transportation accidents or from heart attacks while shoveling snow. Downed powerlines and electricity outages can leave people without heat or in danger of hitting live wires. People exposed to the severe cold can suffer frostbite, hypothermia, and death. Carbon monoxide poisoning can occur when people use natural gas, oil, kerosene, wood, or charcoal stoves improperly to heat their homes or try to stay warm in their stranded vehicles. People are also injured by snowblowers and falling on icy sidewalks and streets. Some people experiencing medical emegencies die when they can't reach healthcare facilities.

In hilly or mountainous areas, an avalanche can occur when the snow starts to melt and becomes unstable. Injuries from an avalanche can include asphyxiation, frostbite, hypothermia, broken bones, and damage to internal organs from being rolled or buried. Avalanches are more common from December to April, but people have died in snowslides throughout the year. These snow events become emergencies when they harm many people and structures.

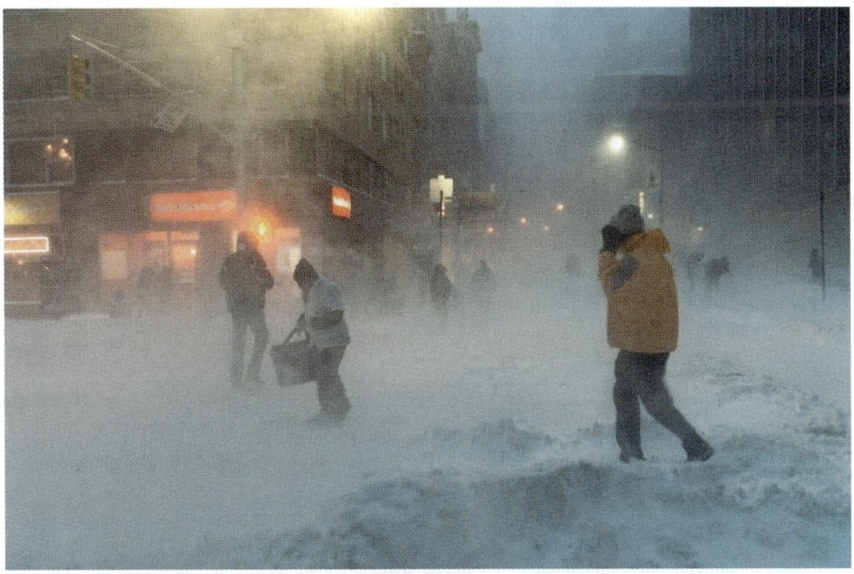

This New York City scene on January 23, 2016 shows how visibility can decrease and snow levels increase. Travel to healthcare facilities may be impossible, and families may be unable to reach their elderly or sick members for basic needs. This winter storm (January 21-29) covered many states and was the biggest blizzard in New York City since 1869. Bus, rail, and elevated subway services, bridges and tunnels were shut down. Three people in New York City died from shoveling snow and three from other causes.

Earthquakes

Expand Your Knowledge

To learn more about earthquakes, watch this National Geographic video: http://EmDPrp2.ParadigmEducation.com/earthquakes-101.

Be Aware

Although most people think of California as "earthquake country," 39 states have active earthquake faults. All health facilities should be aware of the faults that are in their area to assess their risk of earthquakes and know how to prepare.

Earthquakes are produced by major shifts of the earth's crust along inner fracture lines, or faults. As two parts of the crust slide by one another or collide, enormous amounts of energy are released. The energy surges out as waves from a central point, called the epicenter. These seismic waves ripple out and cause the earth and foundations of buildings to shake. Earthquakes can collapse buildings and bridges. Fires erupt when gas lines are broken, sometimes causing explosions. Earthquakes can set off avalanches, flash floods, and **tsunamis** (also known as tidal waves).

Different situations influence the number of people who are injured or die in earthquakes. Some reasons include how close the earthquake is to populated areas, the magnitude (power) of the earthquake, the type of housing in the area where the quake happens, and the time of day that the earthquake occurs.

Survivors often suffer multiple injuries. They may suffer lacerations, fractures, and crush injuries during an earthquake, from the collapse of buildings after the earthquake, or during cleanup activities. People pinned under heavy debris can become dehydrated or unable to take medications for their chronic diseases. Many survivors experience high levels of stress that affects their health.

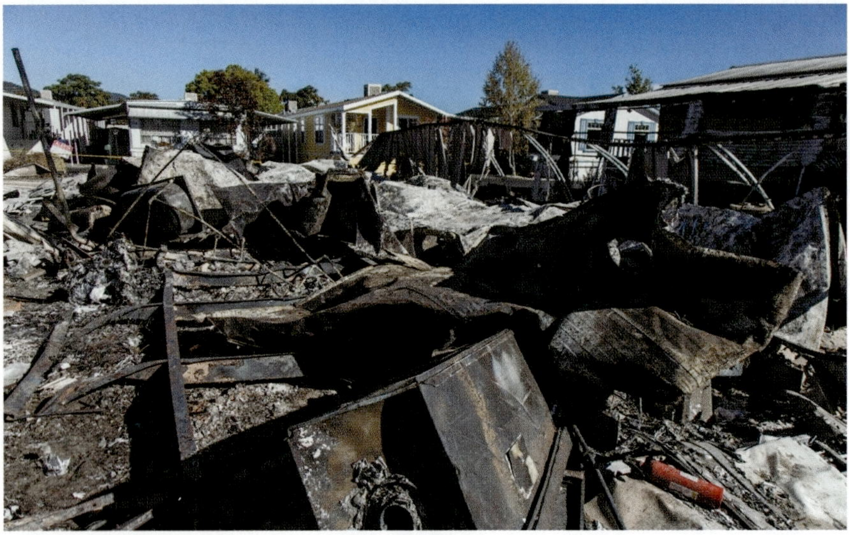

In 2014, Napa and Solano counties in California suffered the largest earthquake in the San Francisco Bay area in 25 years. The earthquake caused a fire in a Napa Valley mobile home park (as seen here), widespread power outages, the damage of 1,600 buildings, roads, and water lines. Two people died, and many were injured. Most injuries occurred while people were cleaning up.

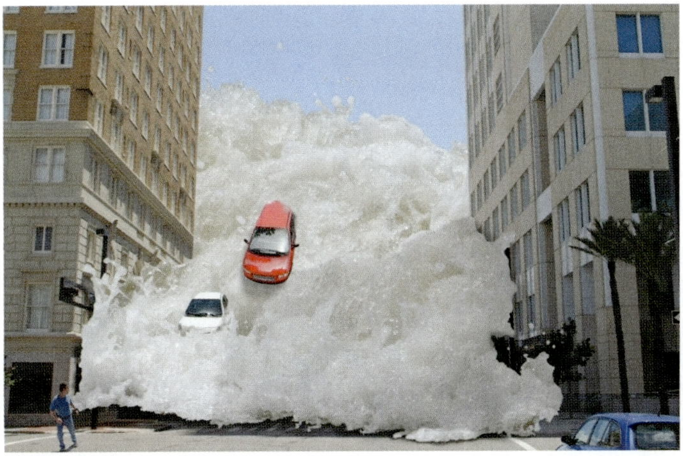

This image shows what can happen in a tsunami. On March 11, 2014, a powerful earthquake struck under the sea 80 miles off Japan's northeastern coast. The earthquake triggered tsunami warnings throughout the Pacific. The tsunami raced outward from the epicenter at nearly 500 miles per hour. Punishing 33 foot waves pushed water as far as 6 miles inland in Japan. The earthquake also sent waves 11 to 12 feet high along the coasts of the islands of Hawaii. Hours later, 9-foot waves crashed on the coasts of California and Oregon.

Tsunamis

Earthquakes can provoke tsunamis, even when the quakes happen in the ocean or in other distant countries across the sea. Tsunamis are a series of powerful waves of water that travel long distances in the ocean and onto the shore. The center of the shaking propels water out in waves. In the deep ocean water, tsunami waves form only a small hump, which generally travels at a very high speed (310 to 620 miles per hour).

When the waves reach shallow water along a coast, the quantity of propelled water swiftly builds up and increases in height, slowing to only 10 miles per hour. These large walls of water can be so powerful that they move everything in their path and cause violent flooding.

To save lives, evacuations to higher ground must begin right after an earthquake hits and there is a threat that a tsunami could form. The US has several warning systems, including sirens, to alert residents about tsunamis in the Pacific Northwest. The US city most often hit by tsunamis is Crescent City, California, and the states most likely to be hit are Hawaii, Alaska, and those of the West Coast, though tsunamis can occur in any coastal area.

After a tsunami, people in the community can become sick because of contaminated water and food supplies. Waterborne diseases, such as diarrheal or fecal-oral diseases can also occur. People can become ill from exposure to animals and mosquitoes or to the bacteria and viruses in the floodwater. People can also acquire tetanus and other infections if they get cut on sharp objects or have open wounds that touch the water.

In addition, when people lose their housing, they are exposed to heat and other environmental hazards if they do not get to shelters. The same problems that happen in other disasters that flood areas, damage homes, and displace people occur and must be addressed by medical teams.

Expand Your Knowledge

To see the real damage of a tsunami, check out the live footage collected on the 2014 Japanese tsunami: http://EmDPrp2.ParadigmEducation.com/tsunami2014.

Web

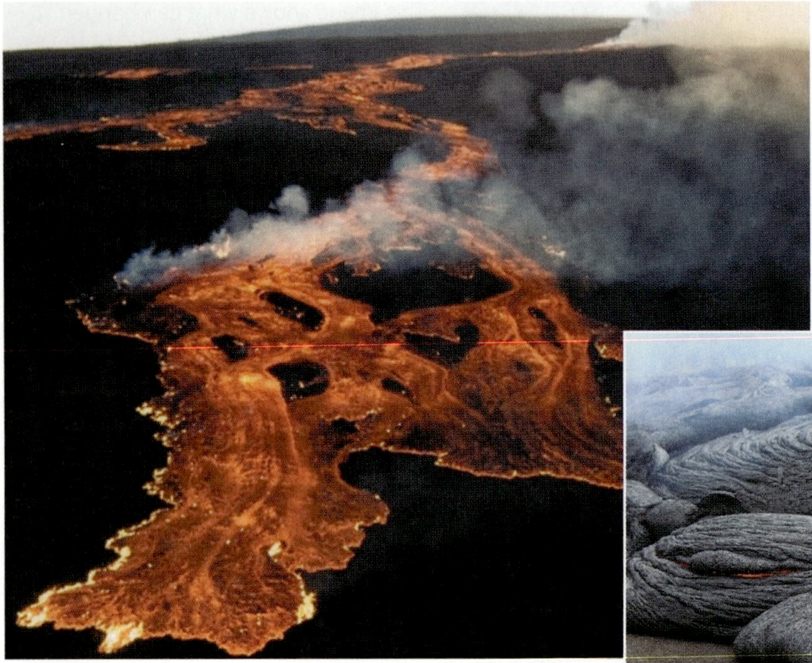

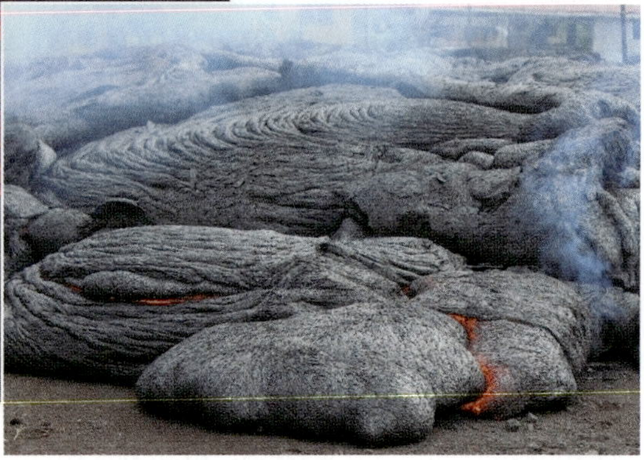

This shows the trail of lava flows in Hawaii after Mauna Loa erupted on March 25, 1984. The lava burned everything its path. The inset shows what cooling lava looks like.

Volcanic Eruptions

A volcano is a mountain or hill that has an inner channel through which molten, or melted, rock can erupt from under the earth's crust. The molten rock is called magma. It is commonly mixed with gases that can build up and put pressure on the earth's crust. When these high pressures can no longer be contained, the gases explode through the crust, expelling large quantities of rocks, fine-grained ash, and lava (crystalized and bubbling magma liquid) into the air. The lava is also extruded, or pushed out like toothpaste, onto the mountainside.

The heat and weight of a flowing lava river can destroy everything in its path, but lava flows usually move slowly enough so that people have time to evacuate safely. The rocks, lava, and ash that rain down from the sky is more dangerous. Many deaths following a volcanic eruption are caused by suffocation from the gases and ash. The ash blasted from the summit can move at hundreds of miles per hour, so it can cause respiratory illness and lung damage to residents far from the site. The ash can also contaminate local and regional drinking water and interfere with electrical power.

People can also be burned by the scalding, hot ash. Ash on the ground can be slippery, so people often are injured by falling. Motor vehicle accidents can occur because of the slippery, fog-like driving conditions.

Expand Your Knowledge

To see images of volcanoes in action, see this National Geographic video: **http://EmDPrp2.ParadigmEducation.com/volcanoes101**.

A Closer Look

Mount St. Helen's Eruption

A small earthquake on March 16, 1980 prompted the eruption of Mount St. Helen's in Washington, and 520 million tons of ash were released. It blocked out the sun in Spokane, and the city went dark. Ash blew 930 miles to central Montana and as far as Minnesota and Oklahoma.

The hot rock and gases melted the mountain's glaciers, causing mud-slides. Forests that were in the path were destroyed. The muddy debris filled up Spirit Lake and caused 600-foot waves to crash onto the other side. Eruptions occurred through summer into the fall. Between 55 and 60 people were killed, and thousands were harmed by the ash and stress.

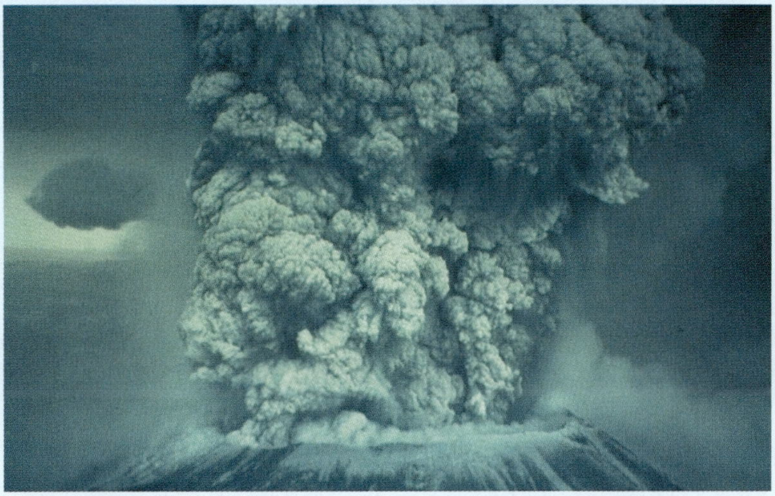

Impacts of Human-Caused Disasters

Beyond natural causes, disasters often also occur due to human accidents and negligence as well as to problems in technology or infrastructure, such as levees, dams, and power plants. Disasters may be intentionally created, as in the case of terrorist attacks. Sometimes a natural event, such as a rainstorm or a flood, becomes a human-caused disaster when the waters mix with toxic chemicals that spread into a community. Accidents or violent attacks that involve chemical, biological, radiological, nuclear, or high-yield explosive substances are referred to as **CBRNE** (or CBRN without explosives). The varied types of human-caused disasters will be explored in this section.

Mass Casualties from Trauma

Accidents or events where many people are injured or killed are known as **mass casualty incidents**. Train crashes and derailments, and airplane crashes are all such disasters. Problems in a community's transportation infrastructure, such as a collapsing bridge or tunnel, can create similar community-wide emergencies. Although infrequent, failing infrastructure like a collapsing bridge or tunnel can result in enough fatalities and serious injuries to test or overwhelm emergency healthcare resources. Since the infrastructure in the US is aging, more emergencies of this type may occur.

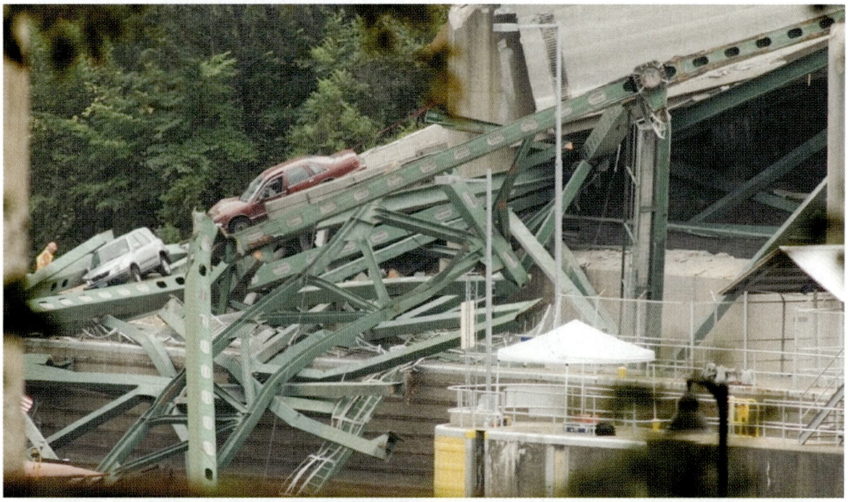

The collapse of the Interstate 35W bridge over the Mississippi River, near downtown Minneapolis, occurred on August 1, 2007. Thirteen people died and approximately 100 were injured in the immediate aftermath of the collapse.

Harmful Chemical Spills and Releases

Accidents, spills, or acts of terrorism that result in the release of dangerous chemicals pose severe threats to human health and the environment. They can leak from industrial plants or from transportation accidents, causing toxic vapors and explosions. Different types of hazardous chemicals have different effects on health. Typically, they cause serious respiratory problems, skin diseases, and burns. If a person is directly exposed to highly toxic chemicals, they can die immediately.

A fire and explosion occurred at the Williams Olefins Plant in Geismar, Louisiana, just south of Baton Rouge, on June 13, 2013. A vapor cloud escaped from a piece of cracked equipment that then ignited, and exploded. Two workers were killed and more than 100 were injured. Health personnel had to treat the victims for heat and chemical injuries. Local authorities ordered people within two miles of the site to close their windows and stay inside. This is called a **shelter-in-place** order.

Polluted water supplies are also human-caused disasters. Severe ongoing public health issues occurred in Flint, Michigan after the municipal authorities decided to use the Flint River as a drinking water source. From the early 1900s, automobile plants had poured industrial waste into the river. In 2014, the river water was treated for human consumption, but it was still smelly and brown coming from the taps. The water also required an additive so it would not cause the pipes to rust when it flowed through. But the city did not add it. Citizens were concerned. Healthcare staff saw rises in numerous health issues in the neighborhoods that had to use the water, including Legionnaires Disease and lead poisoning. Children suffered irreversible damage after unknowingly drinking the water with elevated lead toxins.

A Closer Look

Deepwater Disaster

The Deepwater Horizon oil explosion on April 20, 2010 had the most far-reaching environmental, health, and financial effects of any recent industrial accident. Almost 210 million gallons of oil spilled into the northern Gulf of Mexico when the Deepwater Horizon oil platform exploded, burned, sank, and emitted oil until September. Eleven workers died, and those in boats, ships, and on the coasts were exposed to toxic chemicals. Cleanup workers inhaled fumes from the oil and toxic chemicals used in the cleanup.

These chemical exposures caused many physical problems, including neurological (headache, dizziness), respiratory (cough, wheezing, sore throat), gastrointestinal (nausea, vomiting), cardiac (chest pain, palpitations), skin (rashes, itching, redness), and eye (irritation, blurred vision) issues. Balls of tar washed up on the beaches, making swimming dangerous. People who made a living from catching and selling shrimp and other seafood could not work because they were not allowed in the contaminated water.

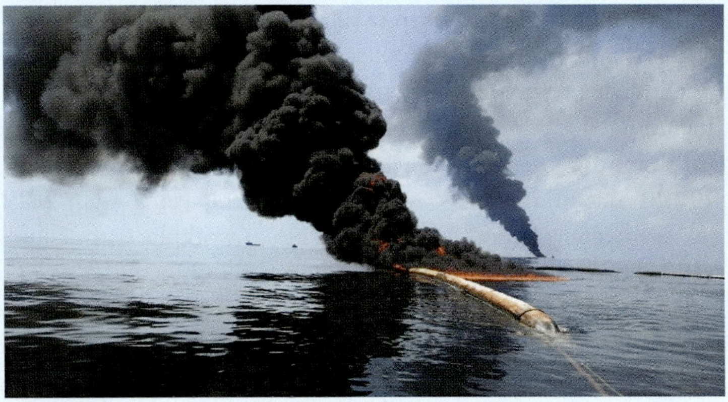

Dark clouds of smoke and fire emerge as oil burns during a controlled fire in the Gulf of Mexico, May 6, 2010. The controlled fire was used to stop the oil spreading from the destroyed Deepwater Horizon offshore drilling unit.

Radiation and Nuclear Accidents

Radiation can leak or explode from an industrial factory or waste products, nuclear power plant, or nuclear weapon. Disaster preparedness training considers radiation from industrial products and waste as one type of emergency and the more concentrated exposure from a nuclear power plant or weapon as another. That is why the CBRNE training addresses chemical, biological, radiological, nuclear, and high-yield explosive agents separately.

Be Aware

Radiation leaks have occurred in the US and around the world. In 2016, it was discovered that the Indian Point Power plant on the Hudson River in New York was leaking radiation into the groundwater.

Symptoms related to radiation exposure depend on the intensity of the exposure and whether it is external or internal. Intense external exposure results in burns. Exposure internally affects cellular structures and can result in cancer. The extent of exposure determines the amount of damage. Small doses can impact the central nervous system. Large doses can lead to death or radiation sickness, with multi-system problems involving the nerves, lungs, and immune system. Radiation sickness decreases protection against infections, which can result in illness and death.

As nuclear power plants age or are decommissioned, nuclear leaks can happen more easily. For instance, in 1979, the reactor at Three Mile Island in Pennsylvania experienced a partial meltdown. In 2017, it was discovered that the cooling canals at the Turkey Point Nuclear Generating Station, south of Miami, have been leaking radioactive water into Biscayne Bay in Biscayne National Park. It is critical that communities be prepared because a nuclear power plant or storage site could be damaged or destroyed by an accident or a terrorist attack.

Terrorist Incidents

Communities also plan for terrorist events. The US Department of Defense defines terrorism as "the unlawful use of violence or threat of violence, often motivated by religious, political, or other ideological beliefs, to instill fear and coerce governments or societies in pursuit of goals that are usually political." Shootings that involve many people can be either a simple crime, where local police conduct the investigation, or an act of terrorism, where federal agencies, including the Federal Bureau of Investigation (FBI), are involved. Sadly, mass shootings have become increasingly frequent across the US. Shooting deaths and injuries have occurred in schools (such as in 2012 at Sandy Hook Elementary School in Connecticut), at workplaces, in churches (more than 20 church shootings have occurred since 1999), and other public places, such as movie theaters and nightclubs.

Terrorist bombings (high-yield explosives) quickly cause many casualties. Without warning, life changes in seconds. The bombings at the Boston Marathon in 2013 and the attacks on the World Trade Center and Pentagon on September 11, 2001 cannot be forgotten. In 2016, 31 people were injured in three separate terrorist bombings in New York City and New Jersey. These events were considered foreign terrorism.

Terrorist attacks can also be accomplished by US citizens, called **domestic terrorism**. In 1995, a domestic terrorist used a truck loaded with explosives to bomb the Alfred P. Murrah Federal Building in Oklahoma City. The bomb destroyed one-third of the building, killing 168 people, including 19 young children in the day-care center. The bombing during the Atlanta Olympics in 1996 was also domestic terrorism.

Responding to any terrorist attack requires an additional level of communication and coordination beyond what's needed for a natural disaster. It involves working with federal investigators and the Department of Homeland Security.

Explosions can injure all parts of the body and cause fractures, hearing problems, and burns. Health personnel can also expect to treat lung injuries, which may result in continual health problems or death. Emergency responders have been injured at incident sites while searching for survivors, so they must be particularly watchful for hazards. Dogs are often used to find bombs to prevent their detonation or buried or trapped victims after disasters strike.

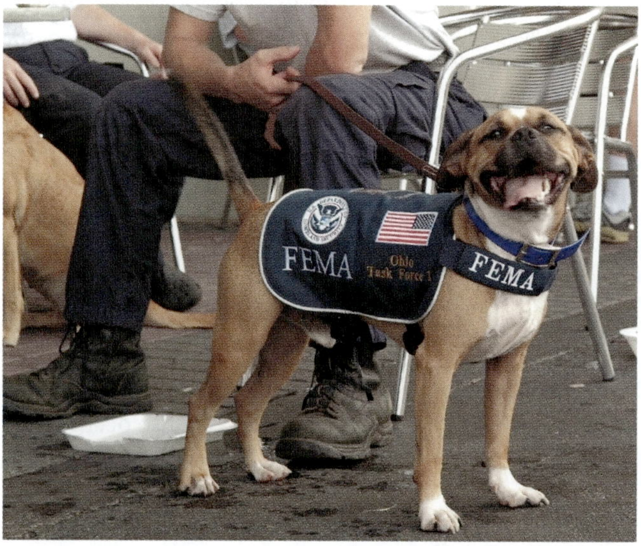

Rescue dog, Buster, of Urban Search and Rescue Ohio Task Force 1, relaxes briefly before being deployed to help in rescue efforts.

Impacts of Infectious Diseases

Infectious diseases may accompany disasters, arise from natural causes, or be deliberately caused by bioterrorism. Infectious diseases can be quickly spread when people are displaced from their homes, staying in crowded shelters, or gathered in close contact in schools, at work, or at public events. The disruption of public utilities and interruption of basic public health services compromises sanitation and hygiene, increasing the risks of infection. Finally, infectious diseases can be spread by plane, train, and bus travel and just daily living. The nation's health protection agency is the **Centers for Disease Control and Prevention (CDC)**. The CDC tracks infectious diseases and works internationally and with states to prevent them from spreading.

Be Aware

An infectious disease for humans is a kind of disease that is transmitted through person-to-person contact or through contact with an infected person's secretions in the air, in water, or on objects.

Emerging Infectious Diseases

Be Aware

Providing bat houses for bats, regularly changing water in birth baths, and getting rid of any standing water in buckets, tires, and other containers around buildings can help reduce mosquito populations. Wearing mosquito repellant can prevent Zika infections and any other disease carried by mosquitoes. Infected patients are advised to get plenty of rest and take medications to reduce pain and inflammation. For more Zika information, go to the CDC website at www.cdc.gov/zika/.

Infectious diseases that were previously unknown in a particular place or appear in a changed and more dangerous form are called **emerging infectious diseases**. For example, the Zika virus, which is a public health concern in the southern US, has been carried by mosquitos in parts of Africa and Asia since 1947. But in 2015, Zika arrived in Brazil and spread rapidly. Zika is transmitted to humans through mosquito bites, sexual relations, blood transfusions, and from mother to child during pregnancy. The exposed child can develop microcephaly (substantially smaller than normal head size) and other defects, or can die before birth. Although most infected adults don't feel very sick, some may later develop Guillain-Barré syndrome, where the immune system attacks the nerves, causing muscle weakness and paralysis. The CDC is working on infection prevention while scientists are seeking a cure and a vaccination to this emerging disease in the US.

Epidemics and Pandemics

Health professionals are always watching out for trends that show an increase in new cases of infectious illnesses. When a highly infectious disease causes people to get sick or die in one area, it is considered an **outbreak**. An **epidemic** occurs when the outbreak spreads to a wider region. This can be due to people having no or low immunity. Epidemics can also occur when healthcare systems are damaged or destroyed, disrupting treatments, and people are unable to get their regular medical care or continue their medications.

Responding to epidemics requires a team of health professionals. They help track cases, isolate suspected patients from other people, and treat those who are ill. With infectious diseases, healthcare workers must be very careful and wear protective equipment. Otherwise, they can become ill and unable to work, making it difficult to provide healthcare for the population.

An epidemic, if not handled effectively, can grow into a **pandemic**, which occurs when a highly infectious disease spreads around the world. The illness travels from country to country, usually through the movement of people who have been infected or through insects carrying the disease. The disease-causing virus or bacteria (or other biological agent) is usually one that people have not yet developed immunity to.

Expand Your Knowledge

For a sense of how epidemiologists investigate disease sources, play the free game from the CDC called "Solve the Outbreak" at http://EmDPrp2.ParadigmEducation.com/solve-outbreak.

A pandemic infection can cause so many illnesses and deaths that it can quickly overwhelm healthcare systems and resources. **Severe acute respiratory syndrome (SARS)** began as an epidemic in Asia and spread to two dozen countries in North America, South America, Europe, and Asia from November 2002 to July 2003. It infected over 8,000 individuals, almost 10% of whom died. Disease detectives, also known as **epidemiologists**, investigate how the disease-causing agent originated and how to stop it. Fortunately, SARS was identified and contained relatively quickly for a pandemic.

Pandemic influenza occurs every three to four decades. An influenza pandemic in 2009 killed almost 580,000 people, mostly in Africa and Southeast Asia. Public health authorities predict that the next influenza pandemic could infect 30% of the US population. Influenza is dangerous because it can cause secondary complications, such as pneumonia, dehydration, and worsening of chronic respiratory and cardiac problems. It is important that healthcare professionals and patients get flu shots every year.

Expand Your Knowledge

Keep an eye on public health disease issues with CDC's Morbidity and Mortality Weekly Report at www.cdc.gov/mmwr/.

Heroes Corner

1918 Spanish Flu Pandemic

The most significant modern pandemic occurred a century ago (January 1918 to December 1920). A virulent influenza strain affected one-third of the world's population. Every continent, except Antarctica had deaths. In the US, a woman remembered that she "lost her uncle to the flu in 1918 on a Friday, her father on a Monday, her mother on Tuesday, a cousin on Thursday, and the family doctor on Friday."

During pandemics and epidemics, healthcare workers and volunteers are the unnamed heroes. In 1918, communities worked together to help the sick. Since the men were serving in World War I, young women carried stretchers with the Red Cross Motor Corps. Others nursed sick patients, taught people about sanitation and preventing illness, tracked the number of individuals who had become ill, and cooked meals. The healthcare workers wore masks and washing their hands regularly to try to prevent getting ill themselves. Ladies' literary clubs sewed the gauze masks for the volunteers.

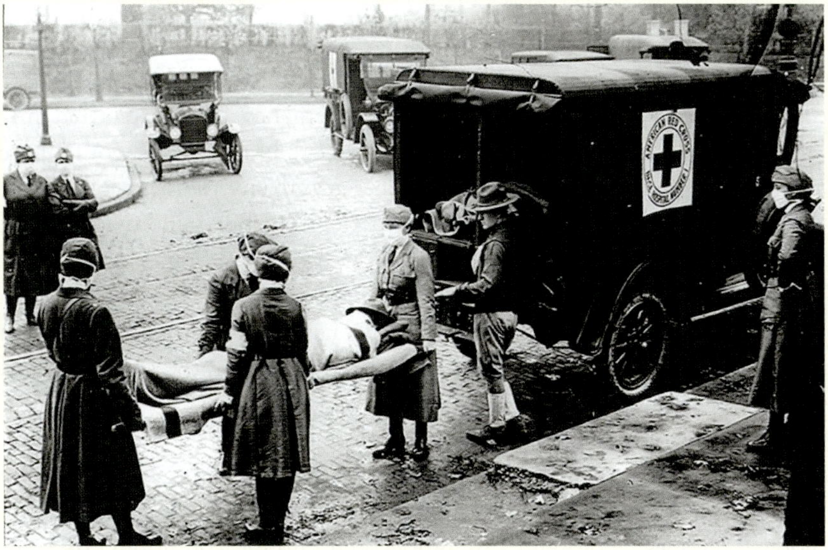

The Motor Corps of the St. Louis chapter of the American Red Cross worked ambulance duty in October 1918.

Web

Bioterrorism **Bioterrorism** is the deliberate release of highly infectious viruses, bacteria, or toxic agents, such as sarin, that can cause illness or death in people, animals, or plants. Biological agents can be spread through the air, through water, or in food. Once contracted, diseases can often be transmitted from person to person. Terrorists can alter the viruses so that they are more likely to cause disease, become resistant to current medicines, or be readily spread into the environment.

The CDC works with state and local public health officials to investigate health effects of bioterrorist incidents. In addition, because of the potential criminal component of bioterrorism, public health professionals may work with the Department of Homeland Security; local, state, and federal law enforcement agencies; the Central Intelligence Agency; and the FBI during the investigation.

The US has experienced incidents of bioterrorism. In 2001, soon after the terrorist attack on the World Trade Center, letters containing spores of anthrax were sent to offices of the news media in New York City and Boca Raton, Florida, and then to several US Senators. Five people were killed and seventeen were infected.

Food has been another target. In 1984, a man who wanted political control of a community in Oregon deliberately used *Salmonella* bacteria to poison the food in salad bars and in salad dressing at ten restaurants, causing 751 people to become ill, and 45 required hospitalization.

Emergency Planning for All Hazards

How can communities prepare for so many different scenarios? All-hazards planning.

Community leaders prepare a general all-hazards disaster plan that describes how they will deal with any emergency or disaster that might occur. They then look at the specific local hazards that could potentially harm people, property, and the natural environment of the area. For example, some places are prone to flooding but seldom experience a blizzard. Tornadoes are common in the Midwest and South but are rare in California, where earthquakes are a serious concern. Planners try to assess the amount of risk of each hazard and plan for any special actions they might have to take in the most likely situations, using the resources, facilities, and personnel at hand.

Communities are required to assess their resources and work with all authorities, businesses, civic groups, and healthcare facilities to be ready for disasters. They seek to protect and treat all citizens: people of all neighborhoods and ages, those with disabilities and chronic conditions, those who struggle with English, and those who lack the resources to prepare their families for disasters. This is known as **whole community preparedness**.

The Roles of Health Professionals

As part of their preparation, communities organize **healthcare coalitions (HCC)** to prepare for and respond to emergencies. The coalitions encompass healthcare facilities and organizations that agree to work together in preparedness planning, prioritizing, and training to be ready to act in a coordinated way in emergency and disaster situations. In addition to hospitals and clinics, these coalitions may include Emergency Medical Services (e.g., ambulances and medevac), hospitals, clinics, ambulatory surgical centers, pharmacies, and private physician practices. Almost 95% of US hospitals participate in an HCC.

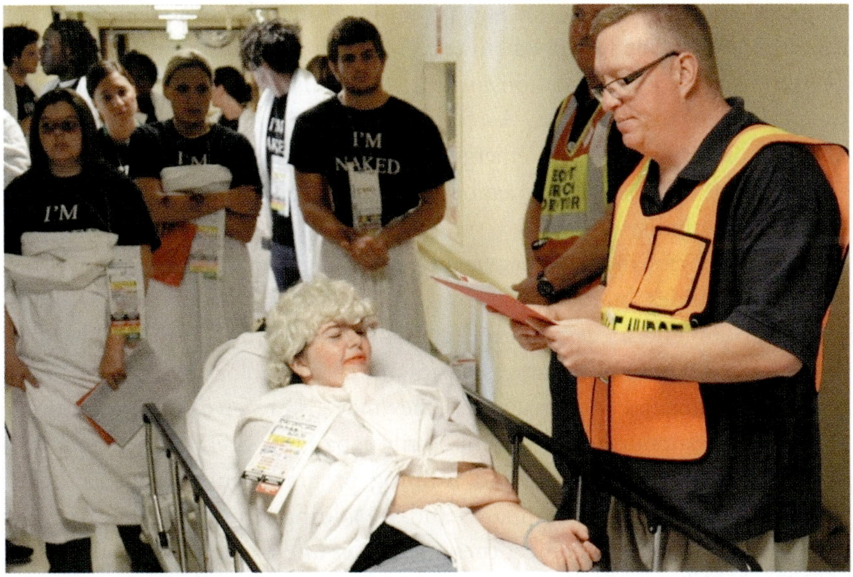

In this preparedness training exercise, hospital staff role-play response to a surge of patients. They are learning what steps different staff members should take and how to receive coordinated direction.

Each healthcare facility must follow the federal preparedness requirements. Seventeen types of facilities, including most of the healthcare organizations that participate in HCCs and long-term care facilities, home health agencies, and providers of outpatient therapy, must comply with the **Emergency Preparedness Rule**. This rule has four requirements:

- An emergency plan
- Emergency policies and procedures
- An emergency communication plan
- Training for and testing of the plan

As facilities plan and train for emergencies and disasters, they need their allied health staff to be knowledgeable and prepared to fill vital roles in these situations. To prepare them and maintain accreditation, all facilities hold emergency drills to practice their response to an emergency.

Scope of Practice and Emerging Expectations

The most obvious healthcare workers needed in an emergency are doctors, nurses, paramedics, and **emergency medical technicians (EMTs)**. Other crucial workers include the many allied health professionals, such as medical assistants, laboratory technicians, pharmacy technicians, and respiratory technicians. Most have basic medical skills that can be of assistance in emergencies. Their contributions are invaluable, particularly when every hand is needed.

When health professionals respond, they each do so within their **scope of practice**. This is the legal and professional definition of their range of expertise and trained responsibilities. A pharmacy technician can be very helpful distributing medications in a shelter or distribution center under the supervision of a pharmacist. A respiratory technician, however, could not dispense prescriptions in an emergency. This would be beyond that professional's scope of practice. Remembering one's scope of practice is critical for maintaining quality of care.

Be Aware

Certified medical assistants, medical laboratory technicians, physician assistants, and pharmacy technicians, among other allied health professionals, all have required standards in emergency and disaster preparedness for certification. Some of these requirements are listed in the eBook's student supplements.

In emergencies and disasters, healthcare professionals carry out their usual job responsibilities, but often they must work faster, harder, and longer. Their work environments are less controlled and more stressful. They may be called upon to work with power outages or unfamiliar technology, fewer tools, and/or less than adequate infrastructure. They may also receive onsite training to assist in other supportive roles, temporarily expanding their scope of practice.

The academic education and training programs for many healthcare professions have adopted standards and are adding required course work to prepare their graduates to meet these new roles and expectations.

Most healthcare professionals are eager to do whatever they can to help in an emergency or disaster. Though responding to an incident is stressful, it is also deeply fulfilling. It demonstrates what it means to be a good citizen and true professional, tested under fire.

By studying and applying the principles discussed in this book, you will build a foundation of knowledge about emergency and disaster response. Through your workplace, you will receive training and participate in drills that are specific to your facility. Continuing education courses on emergency and disaster preparedness are also offered by professional organizations, schools, and volunteer groups. Additionally, look for resources and specialized courses on the Internet and in your community.

Chapter Summary

Emergencies are situations that threaten public safety, health, and welfare. A disaster is an emergency that requires outside assistance from the federal government. As described, the many types of disasters have different causes and effects. Natural disasters are generally caused by weather or geological events. Human-caused disasters result from deliberate acts, poor decisions, or failures in technology or infrastructure. Future disasters may include emerging infectious diseases for which people have little immunity.

All disasters produce both direct and indirect effects. Some effects can be predicted as typical for a specific type of disaster. Others cannot, such as the unique indirect effects, such as winds causing volcano ash to disturb air traffic at a nearby airport slowing aid coming in.

Preparing to respond to these various types of incidents and their effects is called emergency and disaster preparedness. Planning takes an all-hazards approach that can be applied in all types of disasters. Planners also consider likely local hazards. Health professionals work within their scope of practice to provide health care to victims. They need to be prepared to work in unusual circumstances, with fewer technological aids, and under greater stress. But the rewards of helping can provide deep satisfaction.

Additional Resources

To extend the content presented in this chapter, take advantage of the resources available through the chapter's eBook resource links and the end-of-chapter

Key Terms	
all-hazards planning	flash flooding
bioterrorism	healthcare coalitions
disaster	incident
domestic terrorism	mass casualty incident
emergency	natural disaster
emergency and disaster preparedness	nongovernmental organizations
Emergency Preparedness Rule	outbreak
Emergency Medical Service	pandemic
emergency response	scope of practice
emerging infectious disease	shelter-in-place
epidemic	tsunami
epidemiologists	victims
first responders	whole community preparedness

links. These resources include informational supplements and flash cards for terms and abbreviations.

Recognizing Terms

Choose the word or phrase from the list of key terms that best matches each of the following descriptions. Your instructor may ask you to submit your work for grading or may provide you with an answer key for self-assessment.

1. A type of human-caused disaster intended to make people ill ________
2. A contagious illness that is becoming more of a public health problem ________
3. A process that can be applied to a wide range of emergency situations ________
4. When a highly infectious disease spreads around the world ________
5. The people who are injured or become ill as a result of an emergency or disaster ________
6. Disease detectives who investigate how diseases spread from person to person ________
7. Organizations that are not part of government, but they may still provide services ________
8. Readiness by governmental agencies, healthcare systems, community groups, and families take to prevent, respond to, and recover from emergencies ________
9. When healthcare facilities and organizations agree to work together to prepare to respond to emergencies and disasters ________
10. The legal and professional definition of a health professional's responsibilities ________

Reviewing Concepts

Choose the response that best answers the question or completes the sentence. Your instructor may ask you to submit your work for grading or may provide you with an answer key for self-assessment.

1. A recommended general principle for emergency preparedness is to encourage responders
   a. to help outside their scope of practice.
   b. to train for earthquakes.
   c. to be ready to administer vaccines.
   d. to prepare for a range of emergencies.

2. What is an example of a direct impact to a disaster?
   a. People lose their medications.
   b. People need temporary shelter.
   c. People lose their eyeglasses.
   d. People are injured by falling debris.
3. Which disaster occurs more frequently than any other type of disaster?
   a. tornado
   b. flood
   c. hurricane
   d. earthquake
4. One of the most potentially dangerous results of a volcanic eruption in terms of direct injuries and human loss of life is
   a. an earthquake.
   b. an increase in global warming.
   c. a mudflow.
   d. suffocation from gases and ash.
5. A disaster that could be natural or human-made is
   a. an earthquake.
   b. an oil spill.
   c. a wildfire.
   d. a heat wave.
6. Which disaster is most likely to result in radiation exposure?
   a. nuclear power plant explosion
   b. train accident
   c. infrastructure collapse
   d. fire in a chemical-manufacturing plant
7. Which abbreviation can refer to some terrorist incidents?
   a. CBRNE
   b. HCC
   c. SARS
   d. FEMA
8. Which factor may make an influenza pandemic more likely?
   a. Medical records are lost or destroyed.
   b. People have no immunity to the emerging disease.
   c. Many people go to the emergency department for care.
   d. Seasonal weather changes shifts conditions.

9. What is often the first challenge for healthcare workers in an emergency?
   a. analyzing why the emergency occurred
   b. seeking assistance from the federal government
   c. assessing the cost of damages
   d. determining what has happened
10. What are emerging infectious diseases?
    a. diseases that don't affect many people
    b. diseases that can be easily cured
    c. diseases that are new to an area or have changed in the way they spread or how infectious they are
    d. diseases that we know a lot about
11. Whole community preparedness is
    a. being sure that everyone knows everyone in the community.
    b. including children in planning for disasters.
    c. working with everyone to protect people of all neighborhoods and ages.
    d. having a translator at every planning meeting.
12. What are ways that you can expand your knowledge about preparedness?
    a. training and drills at work
    b. continuing education courses offered by professional organizations and schools
    c. courses on the Internet and in your local healthcare facility and community
    d. All of the answers are correct.
13. What kinds of diseases can people develop from sewage in a flood?
    a. respiratory
    b. gastro-intestinal and skin diseases
    c. cardiac
    d. neurological
14. What is a public health problem that occurs in homes when flood-waters recede?
    a. Furniture has moved around.
    b. People can't find important papers.
    c. Mold develops.
    d. It takes too long to clean up the mess.

15. Why do many people die in a hurricane?
    a. Their cell phones stop working.
    b. They don't evacuate.
    c. They run out of food and water.
    d. They catch a cold from being wet.

Exploring Emergency Preparedness Issues

Complete the following activities to further explore the concepts found in this chapter. Your instructor may ask you to submit your work for grading or may provide you with guidance for self-assessment.

1. Visit NOAA's National Weather Service web page (http://www.nws.noaa.gov/view/largemap.php), to see the active watch, warnings advisories, and short term forecasts.
2. Go to the CDC's *Morbidity and Mortality Weekly Report* at www.cdc.gov/mmwr/. Type "disasters" in the box next to MMWR Search. Find one case report about a disaster that occurred in your region of the country. Describe the circumstances of that disaster and its impact on the community. What were the health impacts? Describe how your profession would be involved in caring for victims. Summarize this information in a one- to two-page report.

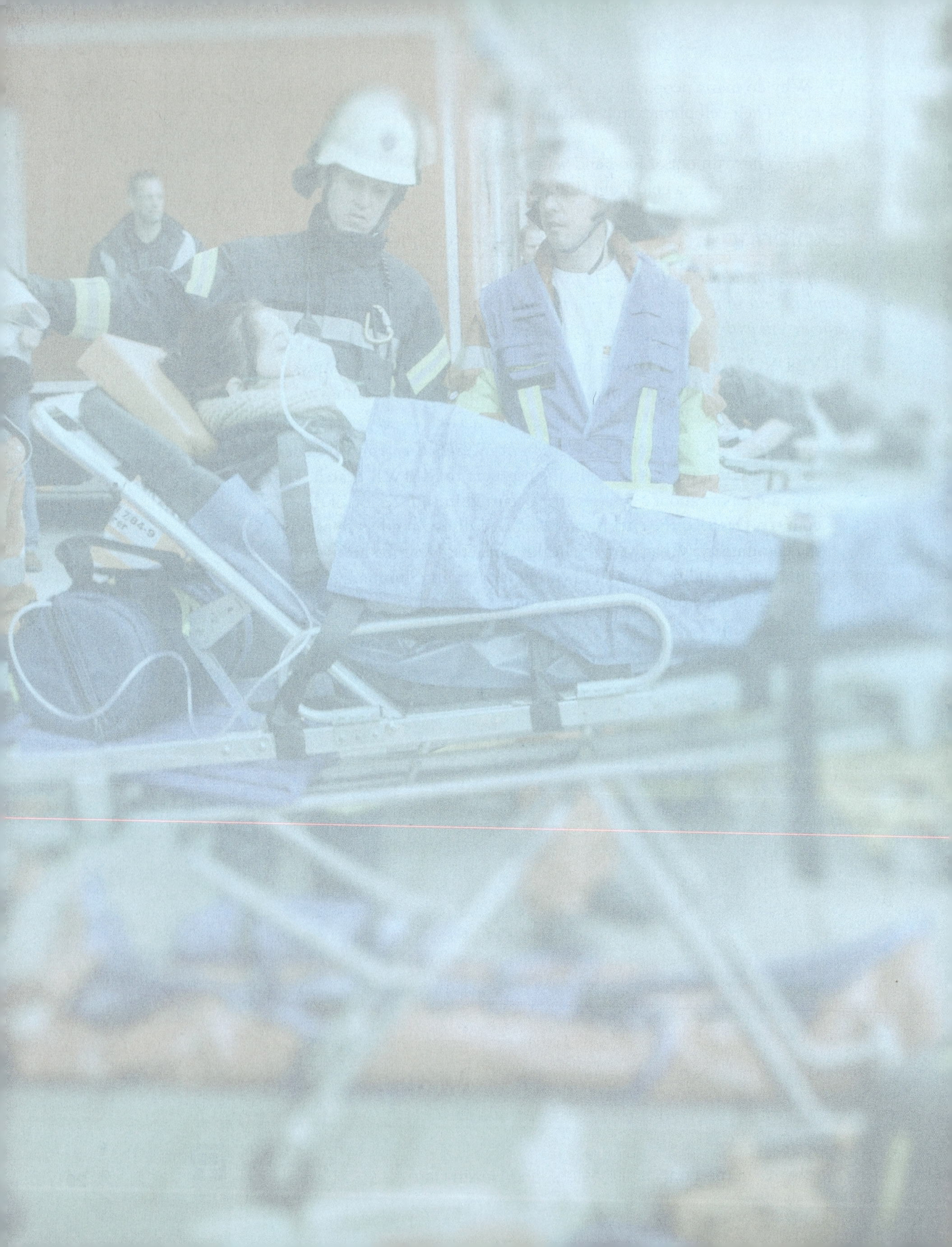

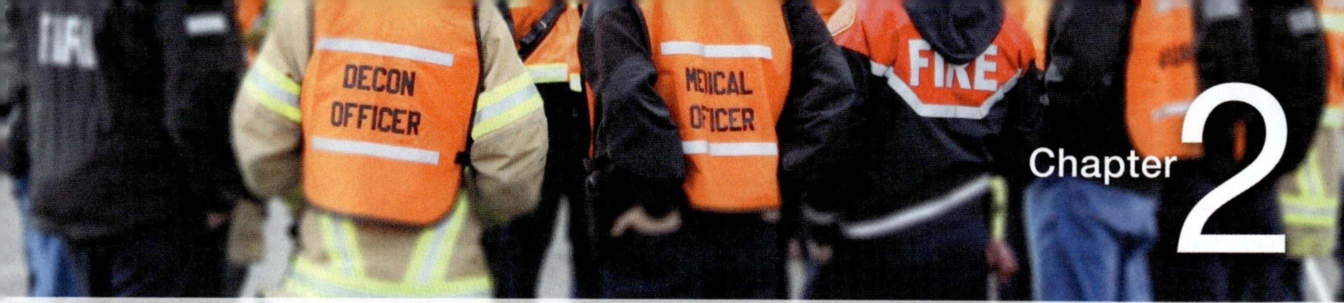

Chapter 2

Emergency and Disaster Planning and Management

What You Will Learn

- The four phases of comprehensive emergency management
- The federal guidance provided by the National Response Framework and the National Incident Management System
- How the Incident Command System clarifies roles and authority in a response
- The role of a local emergency management agency
- How a disaster requiring federal assistance is declared and what federal resources for health care are deployed, including the National Disaster Medical System
- How nongovernmental resources and groups fit into emergency and disaster response

Who oversees planning for emergencies? When a disaster strikes, who organizes and directs the response? The officials leading a community's planning and response are always the local government and emergency management authorities with other agencies in the community. All US communities and responders follow the same emergency management systems and principles. In this way, a diverse group of local governments, varied government agencies, healthcare facilities, and nongovernmental organizations can work together effectively. Understanding how these nationwide management systems work will help you see the big picture and your place in it.

Comprehensive Emergency Management

To adequately respond to disasters, planners need to consider many levels of concern. Authorities in federal, state, county, tribal, and local government agencies, businesses, and healthcare facilities go through stages of planning. As noted in Chapter 1, communities begin by preparing an all-hazards plan that addresses issues common to every emergency. Communities then need to plan for the specific emergencies and disasters that are most likely to occur in their area or have already occurred. They determine ways to prevent these most probable emergencies and disasters or reduce the effects if they do occur.

The next level of preparation is operational planning: How does the community inform, train, activate, and put all available responders and resources to proper use for effective response? How do they pull together resources within the community and activate them when needed? The planners need to set strategic goals for what they want to accomplish in each level of the response.

Finally, once an emergency or disaster has occurred, how do responders act in a coordinated manner, and how does the local government help the community and people return to normal living?

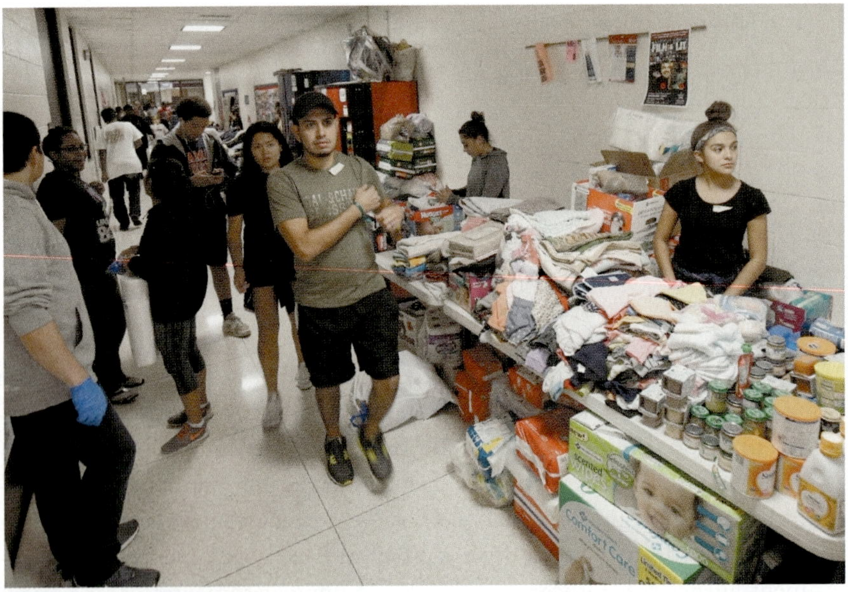

Community groups in Houston donated supplies to the Lone Star College North Harris temporary shelter for evacuees of Hurricane Harvey in August, 2017.

Key Acronyms	
ASPR	Assistant Secretary for Preparedness and Response
CDP	Center for Domestic Preparedness
CERT	Community Emergency Response Team
DHS	Department of Homeland Security
DMAT	Disaster Medical Assistance Team
DMORT	Disaster Mortuary Operational Response Team
DOH	Department of Health (local, county, and state)
EMI	Emergency Management Institute
EOC	emergency operations center
EOP	emergency operations plan
HHS	Department of Health and Human Services
ICS	Incident Command System
LEMA	Local Emergency Management Agency
MRC	Medical Reserve Corps
NDMS	National Disaster Medical System
NIMS	National Incident Management System
NRF	National Response Framework
NVRT	National Veterinary Response Team
OEM	Office of Emergency Management
POD	Point of Distribution
TCCT	Trauma and Critical Care Team
THIRA	Threat and Hazard Identification and Risk Assessment
VOAD	Voluntary Organizations Active in Disaster

To prepare on all these levels, planners use a four-phase approach known as **comprehensive emergency management**. The phases include:

- Prevention and Mitigations of Risks
- Preparedness
- Response
- Recovery

Actions taken in the prevention/mitigation and preparedness phases usually occur before an incident, whereas actions taken in response and recovery occur during and after.

The Phases of Comprehensive Emergency Management

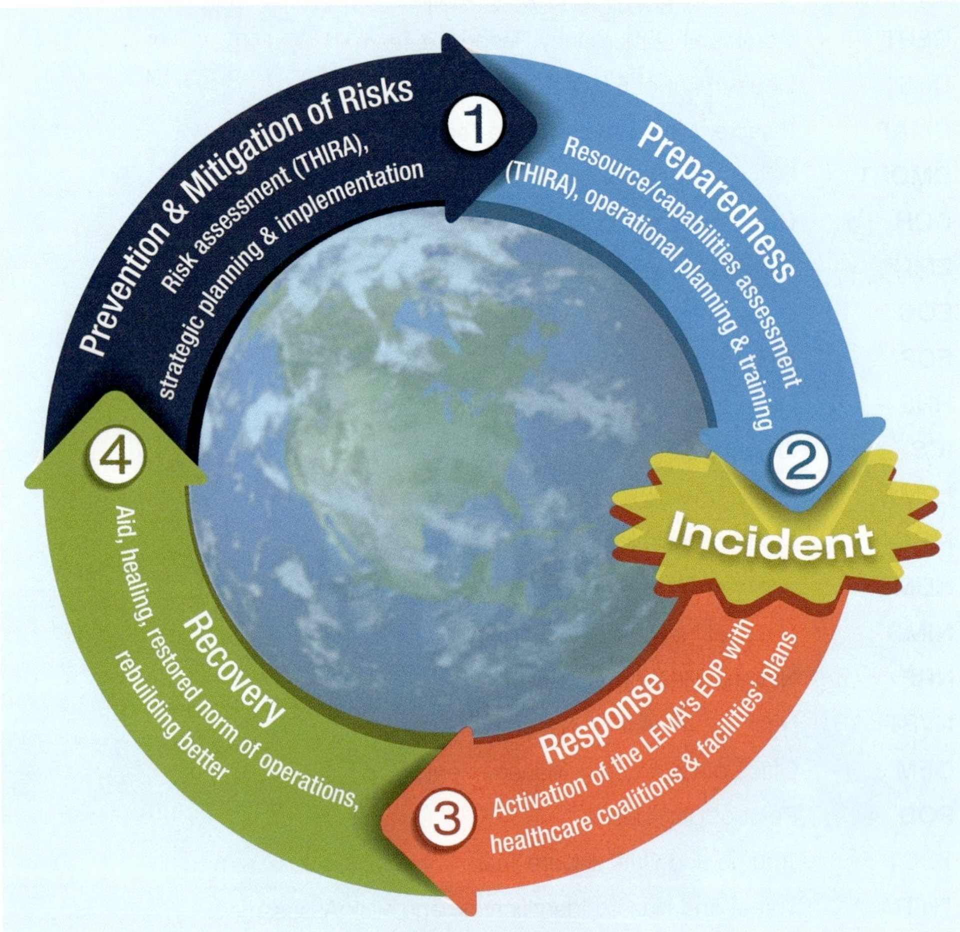
1
Prevention & Mitigation of Risks
Risk assessment (THIRA), strategic planning & implementation
2
Preparedness
Resource/capabilities assessment (THIRA), operational planning & training
Incident
3
Response
Activation of the LEMA's EOP with healthcare coalitions & facilities' plans
4
Recovery
Aid, healing, restored norm of operations, rebuilding better

The process starts with assessing potential hazards and finding ways to prevent damage. Then leaders make operational plans and prepare the staff and public through education, training, and drills. Recovery involves repairing any damage and can include changing infrastructure or processes to reduce or eliminate future similar risks.

Prevention and Mitigation of Risks

The first stage involves the crucial step of assessing the potential risks. Planners use the **Threat and Hazard Identification and Risk Assessment, (THIRA)**, to identify the specific hazards that have harmed people, property, or the environment within their jurisdiction or may in the future.

The communities, county, and state then look for solutions to prevent or minimize harm that could occur from those hazards. This might include building new structures or improving old ones. This is called **mitigation**, or reduction, of risks or potential damage. A Florida community might reinforce storm levees and change zoning to stop additional building in areas prone to flooding. The community would also develop a plan to evacuate citizens in case the mitigation efforts fail.

Preparedness

The **preparedness** phase focuses on getting everything ready for immediate activation if any hazard occurs, with a special emphasis on the identified risks. All the operational planning, education, and training for readiness happens in this phase. Preparedness includes the following:

- Identifying the goals and tasks needed to respond to identified risks and the personnel that would be needed—the second step of THIRA.
- Establishing a place for an **Emergency Operations Center (EOC)** where community-based emergency management decisions can be made
- Developing communications and warning systems within the local government and community and with others who respond on the local, state, and federal level.
- Organizing available resources and deciding on the delegation of authority and responsibilities.
- Organizing key personnel, equipment, and supplies so that they can be accessed quickly.

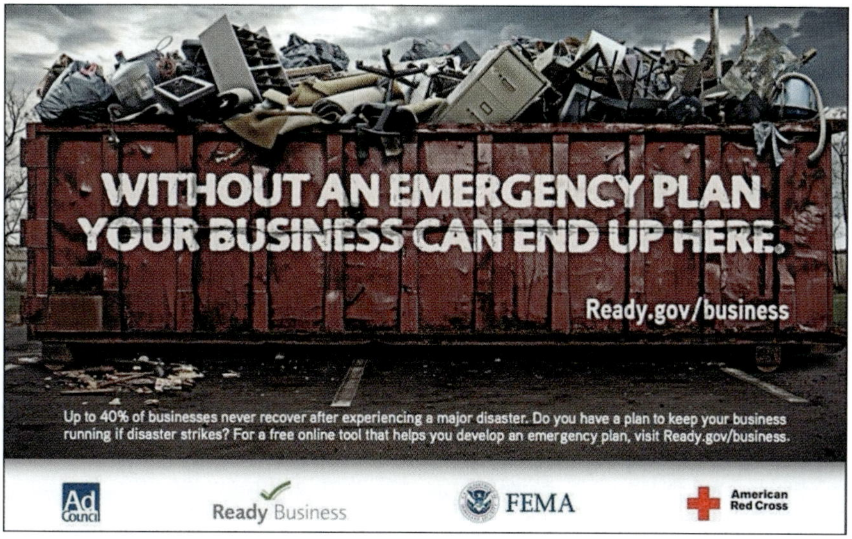
WITHOUT AN EMERGENCY PLAN
YOUR BUSINESS CAN END UP HERE.
Ready.gov/business
Up to 40% of businesses never recover after experiencing a major disaster. Do you have a plan to keep your business running if disaster strikes? For a free online tool that helps you develop an emergency plan, visit Ready.gov/business.
Ad Council
Ready Business
FEMA
American Red Cross

FEMA provides guidance to help prepare the whole community, including businesses, for emergencies and disasters.

- Creating evacuation plans to get citizens out of harm's way.
- Training personnel to follow the response plans so they are ready.
- Conducting **emergency exercises**—drills to test the plans.
- Stockpiling supplies, food, water, and other needed elements.
- Developing agreements with neighboring communities or institutions that could quickly provide personnel, equipment, and materials, known as **mutual aid**.

Response

The term **response** refers to immediate actions to save lives, protect property and the environment, and meet basic human needs. The response phase occurs immediately before, during, or after the incident. It includes the first responders and then the healthcare system and all other response resources, determined by the scope of the event.

With weather disasters, such as hurricanes, communities usually receive advance warning, and they can begin working on an early response. When in the direct path of a dangerous storm, communities and healthcare facilities consider implementing evacuation plans. They may need to alert and move residents and patients to safety and set up ways to provide sufficient medical care. Safety and response information has to be communicated through many channels to reassure the public and direct people in next steps and what to expect. Food, water, shelter, and medical assistance should be readied for efficient and fair distribution to evacuees at accessible locations. Once the hurricane hits, the developed action plans are then activated at affected locations, such as in flooded neighborhoods.

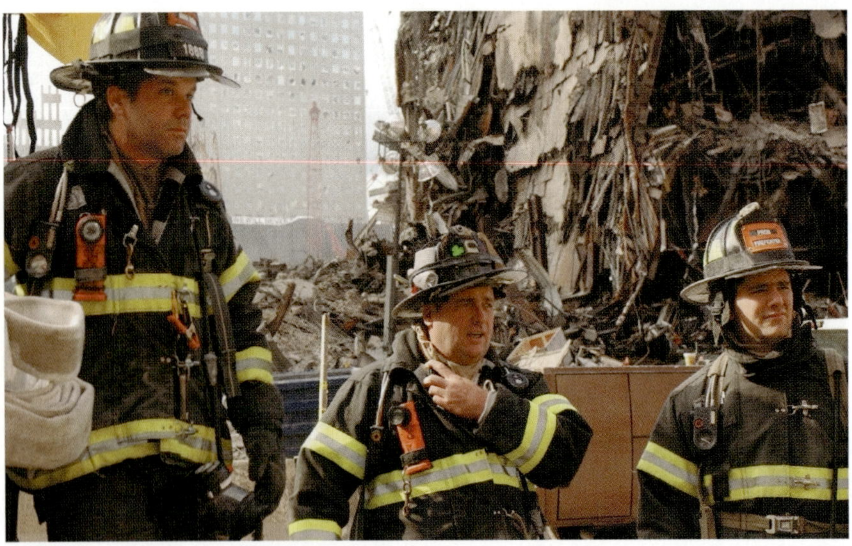

Local personnel are the first to respond to emergencies. Local firefighters are shown in the wreckage of the World Trade Center in September 2001.

In all emergencies or disasters, response begins with the first responders helping victims at the incident site, who have often been dispatched there by a 9-1-1 call service operator. The operator has been specially trained to alert the proper responders and authorities. One such responder is the Emergency Medical Service. Recall that EMS is a local organization that provides emergency medical care at an incident scene and rapid transportation to a hospital emergency department.

While the police, firefighters, and/or EMS are responding on the scene, the local authorities are activating their operational plans and coordinating the larger community response. They will oversee the police action and other law enforcement, work with the healthcare facilities, implement evacuation plans, set up victim assistance, and engage other partners, depending on the nature and scope of the emergency or disaster.

Be Aware

The emergency medical technicians (EMTs) and paramedics follow protocols dictated by a supervising physician.

Recovery

The **recovery** phase includes activities and programs that help a community and victims return to normal or to what may be called a "new normal."

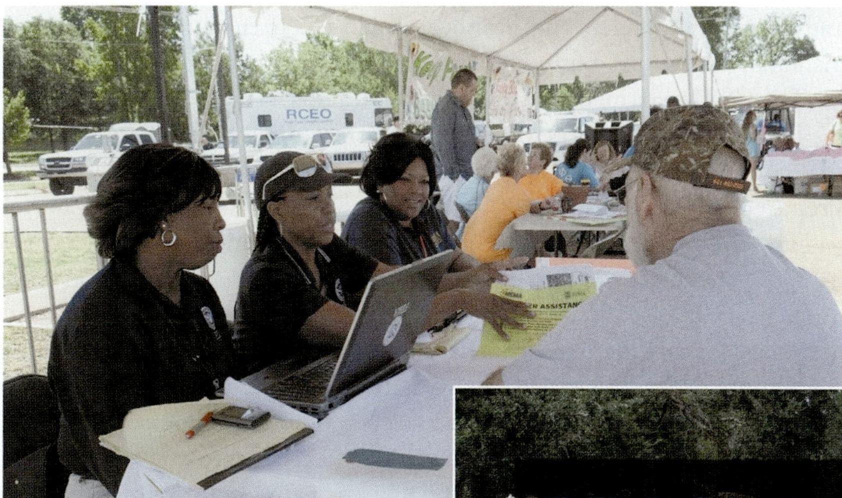
RCEO

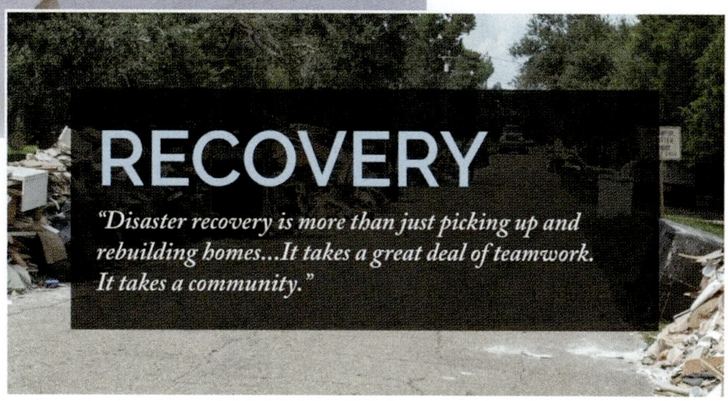
RECOVERY
"Disaster recovery is more than just picking up and rebuilding homes...It takes a great deal of teamwork. It takes a community."

At the Pearl Day Festival in Pearl, Mississippi, in May 2014, FEMA and the Mississippi Emergency Management Agency (MEMA) team up to talk to disaster victims and show them how to apply for federal assistance to recover from damage from recent storms, tornadoes, and flooding. This inset is from FEMA's blog on the third phase of comprehensive emergency management.

Expand Your Knowledge

In counties often hit by disasters, nonprofit organizations quickly organize to help community, faith, civic, and business groups work together with local authorities for disaster planning, response, and recovery. In Florida, there is Be Ready Alliance Coordinating for Emergencies (BRACE). BRACE has a seat in the Escambia County Emergency Operations Center for when emergencies and disasters hit. Explore this example at http://EmDPrp2.ParadigmEducation.com/BRACE.

During recovery, health professionals may be involved in replacing lost medications and delivering medical care in places where healthcare facilities have been destroyed or damaged. It is essential to rebuild destroyed homes and businesses. Helping people grieve and seek out assistance, and repairing hospitals are all part of recovery. Many business, civic, and religious organizations get involved. Rebuilding is an opportunity to improve the structures in a community to help prevent or reduce the destruction of future disasters.

Federal Resources for Comprehensive Emergency Management

The US **Department of Homeland Security (DHS)** is the federal agency in charge of ensuring national safety and promoting comprehensive emergency management. Within this department is the Federal Emergency Management Agency (FEMA). It is the lead federal agency to guide and assist the nation in this area, and it provides resources for this comprehensive planning and management approach. FEMA sets up guidelines and training for leaders in federal, state, county, tribal, and local government agencies; and for first responders and healthcare facilities. It encourages nongovernmental organizations, businesses, and citizens to prepare in similar ways.

The US **Department of Health and Human Services (HHS)** addresses the health-related aspects of emergency and disaster preparedness and response. Within the HHS are the office of the **Assistant Secretary for Preparedness and Response (ASPR)** and the Centers for Disease Control and Prevention (CDC). Both agencies incorporate comprehensive emergency management into their activities, providing guidance and resouces in their different areas of expertise. The ASPR helps state and local agencies and healthcare systems prepare for and respond to the medical needs of an affected community or area. The CDC assists state, county, and local **Departments of Health (DOH)** in infectious disease prevention and response, public health monitoring, citizen awareness, and medical laboratory resources. (The distinct roles of the ASPR and the CDC in assisting healthcare facilities in emergency response and management will be explained in greater depth later in this chapter and in Chapter 3).

National Response Framework

To provide communities and states national direction for the preparation and response to all hazards, the DHS created the National Response Framework (NRF) and the National Incident Management System (NIMS).

The **National Response Framework (NRF)** describes how the federal government organizes itself and plans for disasters, and it provides guidelines for other levels of government and responding organizations to do the same. The NRF is based on the principle that the whole community, with all its different stakeholders and citizens, needs to work together to help everyone prepare for disasters. The NRF supplies planning documents for each of the four phases of comprehensive emergency management.

With the planning documents, state, county, tribal, and local departments of emergency and disaster management can go through the planning processes and organize response strategies in a unified manner with varied governmental and community partners. The NRF helps leaders and groups develop all-hazard emergency plans and specific hazard response plans that are flexible, adaptable, and **scalable** (adjustable to fit the size of the event).

The National Incident Management System

During an emergency or disaster, it is not efficient if responders at any level receive different instructions about what they should do from multiple people in charge. To prevent this problem, the DHS established a command structure model. It is called the **National Incident Management System (NIMS)**. The NIMS provides an operational template for communities to organize themselves and coordinate their response activities in a similar manner. The NIMS accomplishes the following:

- Provides a delineated chain of command called the **Incident Command System (ICS)**.
- Describes how those managing the response delegate tasks from commander to responder and to working groups, with outlined authority and duties for coordinated operational management.
- Establishes standard procedures for managing resources and facilitating coordination that everyone follows when an incident occurs.
- Establishes common principles and terminology so that every responder involved will understand how the affected community deals with the incident.

Like the planning documents of the NRF, the ICS structure is also flexible, adaptable, and scalable so that it may be used for all incidents, large and small. The size of the ICS and the type of personnel involved can be adjusted to the size, magnitude, and special situations of the incident.

The ICS's top-down chain of command has a single person in charge who gives orders. The **incident commander** has the overall responsibility for managing the response within his or her level of authority—overall management or on-site incident management. With input from others, he or she establishes response goals (such as rescuing people trapped in rubble following an earthquake), makes plans for accomplishing the goals, assigns

Be Aware

During the phases of response and recovery, local authorities follow an ICS modeled on the NIMS for making decisions and deploying resources. They meet at the designated EOC. First responders focus on coordinating the actions at the scene of the disaster. The incident commander designates a place where the incident commander and others meet to discuss how the response is going and decide on next actions. It is called the **incident command center**.

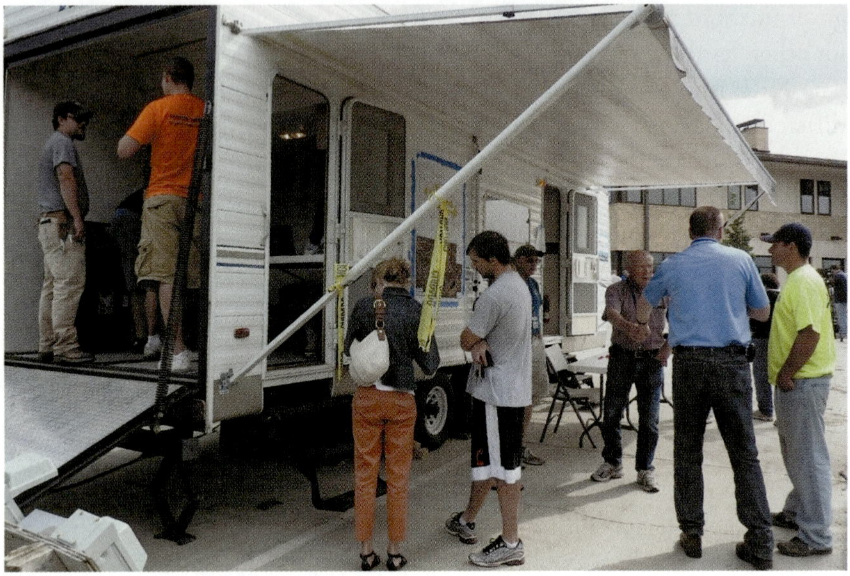

After Missouri River flooding in June 2011, the incident command center of North Sioux City set up an informational trailer. Citizens needed to go there to apply for identification cards to re-enter the flooded area to check their homes for damage.

the specific tasks to the proper personnel trained to accomplish the goals, and prioritizes response activities (such as the on-site decision of rescuing people or clearing debris). The ICS model eliminates any confusion because it makes clear whom everyone reports to and whose orders they must follow.

When the response to a disaster involves more than one community or agency, a **unified command** will be employed. A unified command occurs when all agencies with responsibility for handling the incident work together to establish and implement a single, coordinated plan. Together they decide on a common set of objectives, plan jointly for operational activities, and maximize resources. The command often adapts pre-established all-hazards and specific disaster plans to the circumstances of a particular incident.

The command oversees four working groups:

- **Planning Group**—gathers, processes, and analyzes ongoing information to plan the most effective response with the available resources, communicating the actions needed to meet the strategic objectives to the commander(s)
- **Operations Group**—carries out directives necessary to achieve the objectives; for example, caring for victims of a fire or setting up safety zones around the building
- **Logistics Group**—provides transportation, supplies, equipment maintenance, fuel, food services, communications, information technology support, and medical services for emergency responders
- **Finance and Administration Group**—tracks costs and addresses financial issues, including reimbursement and claims

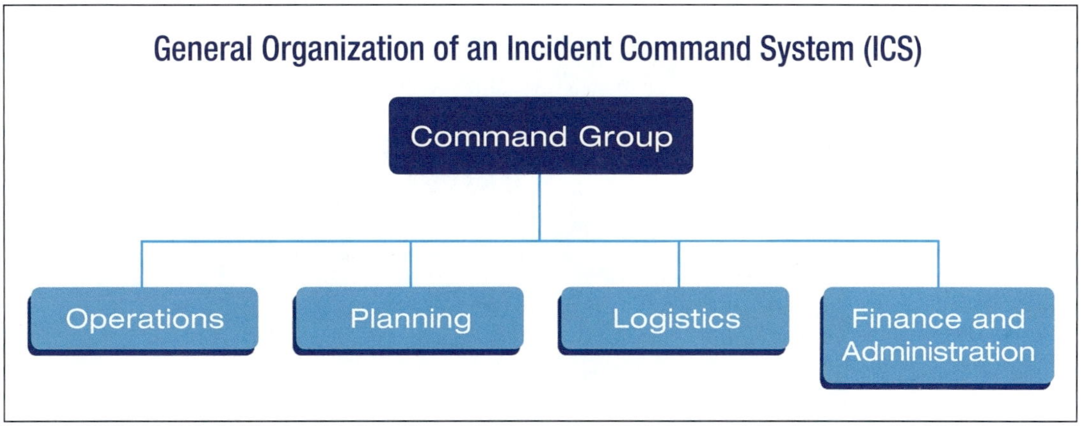

Each ICS is structured so that any of these four groups can be activated or not, depending on the needs of the emergency or disaster. The ICS structure is used at different levels to manage both day-to-day emergencies, such as building fires, and the responses to disasters, such as the terrorist attack on the World Trade Center or the Boston Marathon bombings. The incident commander will delegate the responsibilities of the needed groups.

Using the ICS model, every level of leadership—whether in a city, state, or federal agency, healthcare facility, nongovernmental organization or first responder group—can plan for and manage emergencies and disasters. The ICS of each responding organization is focused only on the goals and tasks required where it is stationed. Healthcare facilities and departments of health use their own form of ICS to organize the response within their facilities or department. (This will be described more in Chapter 3.)

Federal Training in NRF, NIMS, and Response

Effectively organizing a whole community response is complex and difficult. FEMA offers workshops, conferences, and online courses to train local authorities, healthcare facilities, and other responding partners in applying the NRF and NIMS. Participating groups and leaders learn how to go through the processes of comprehensive emergency planning, set up an ICS, and respond effectively to all hazards.

The **Emergency Management Institute (EMI)**, in Emmitsburg, Maryland, teaches comprehensive management principles and how ICS is structured. The **Center for Domestic Preparedness (CDP)**, in Anniston, Alabama, provides hands-on training for all-hazards preparedness to leaders of healthcare facilities alongside EMS, firefighters, law enforcement, public health, and public workers.

Expand Your Knowledge

If you would like to learn more about emergency and disaster preparedness, you can consider free online courses from the EMI. You can view classes and how to quality for enrollment at **https://training.fema.gov/is/**

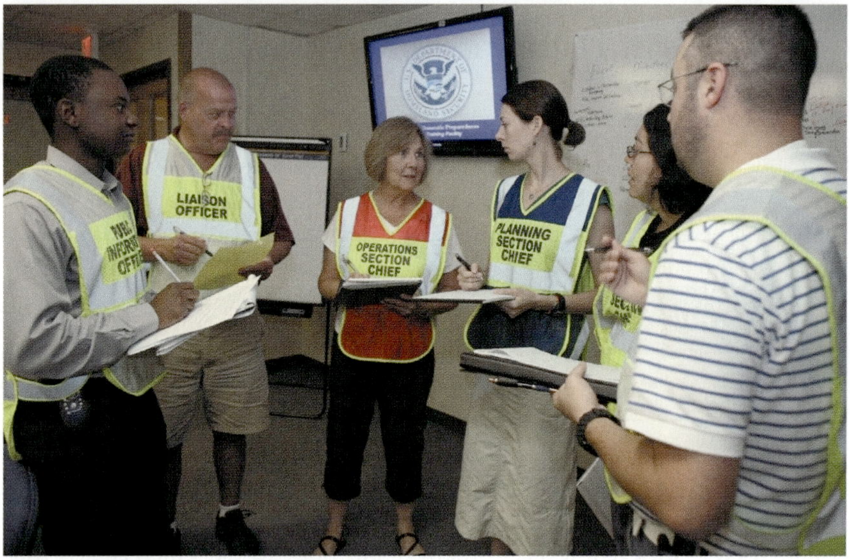

A Colorado Hospital Association team goes through an all-hazards training exercise at the Center for Domestic Preparedness (CDP) in Anniston, Alabama.

Now that we know the federal framework and structure for preparedness and organized response, let's look at how the local level works.

Local Management and Response

Within each community, there is a governmental office or council in charge of emergency and disaster preparedness and response. It is designated as the Local Emergency Management Authority or **Local Emergency Management Agency (LEMA)**. This group establishes its ICS, its EOC, and its working groups. Counties and large metropolitan areas call their LEMA the **Office of Emergency Management (OEM)** and have a professional emergency manager.

In a small community, the LEMA may be a special committee including representatives from the police, firefighters, and EMS. The chief of police or the local public safety official may be the head of the LEMA. During an emergency, the LEMA reports to the mayor or city manager. Oftentimes, the county OEM, which has more resources, becomes the LEMA.

Volunteer groups and local hospitals often plan for emergencies with the LEMA. Using a whole-community approach, the local authorities develop an all-hazards **emergency operations plan (EOP)**. The EOP designates who will be in charge and who will coordinate the public and private efforts, including those of the healthcare coalitions, facilities, and professionals.

The number of agencies involved in the EOP and the degree of preparations vary by the size of the community, resources available, and scope of the potential emergencies or disasters. The plan also determines particular preparation activities, such as taking inventories of equipment and supplies, training staff, and running drills. As part of the EOP, the LEMA works out agreements with other communities for mutual aid. Any personnel, equipment, and other supplies to be provided are considered **assets**.

During any incident, the local government maintains control of all assets regardless of their source (from another community, the state, or federal government). The LEMA works with state and federal agencies in deciding how assets will be used in the response and recovery efforts. For any public health concerns, the local, county, or state DOH often sends one of its health professionals to serve as the liaison with the LEMA.

Even in disasters where federal resources are requested, the local government is still in charge of the response to an emergency or disaster. For example, during and after the 2001 World Trade Center attacks, New York City was still in charge of the response and delivery of services, even though FEMA and other federal and state agencies (including the US military and National Guard), and other responders were called in for assistance.

Incident Command Systems at Work

When the first responders arrive at an emergency or disaster scene, the on-site incident commander is the most senior person. The incident commander is responsible for assessing the situation and directing the response. He or she

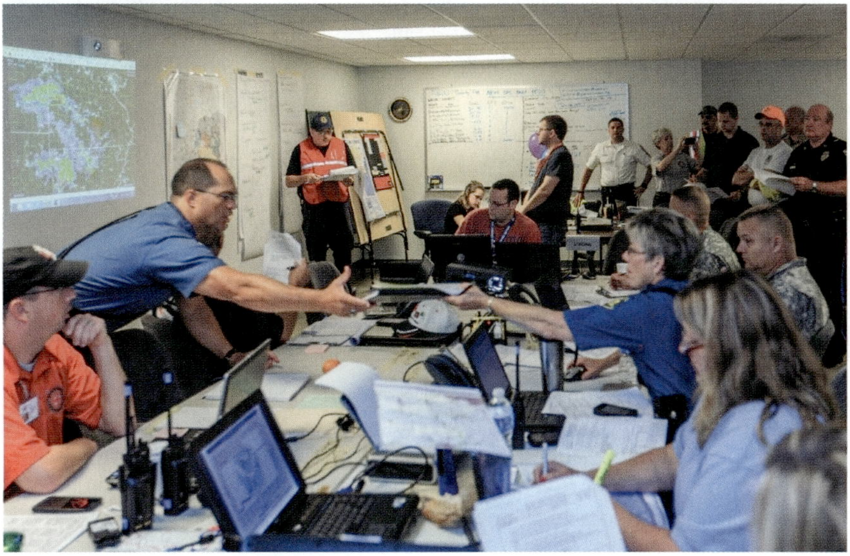

This is an EOC in action in Pulaski County, Missouri, responding to flooding in Waynesville in August 2013.

communicates the status of the response to the local authorities who then oversee the community response. The on-site incident command is transferred to more senior officials as they arrive.

In complex events, such as the World Trade Center attacks, several professionals usually direct the response together. Each is in charge of a particular workforce that joins efforts in a coordinated plan, using the unified command model.

The local authorities at their EOC activate their EOP, coordinate activities and communicate to the public and other levels of government. The EOC of the LEMA may be located at common community places, such as the police station, city hall, or in the OEM (if the community has one).

For public health emergencies, such as when infectious disease is spreading in a community, the local or county Department of Health is in charge. The DOH sets up an incident command center at its offices to coordinate with local healthcare facilities, community providers, the state DOH, and the CDC.

Local Assistance for Victims

During and right after an emergency and disaster, citizens may have the need for food, water, and other supplies. The local authorities, with the county or state OEM, set up **Point of Distribution (POD)** sites. These PODS should

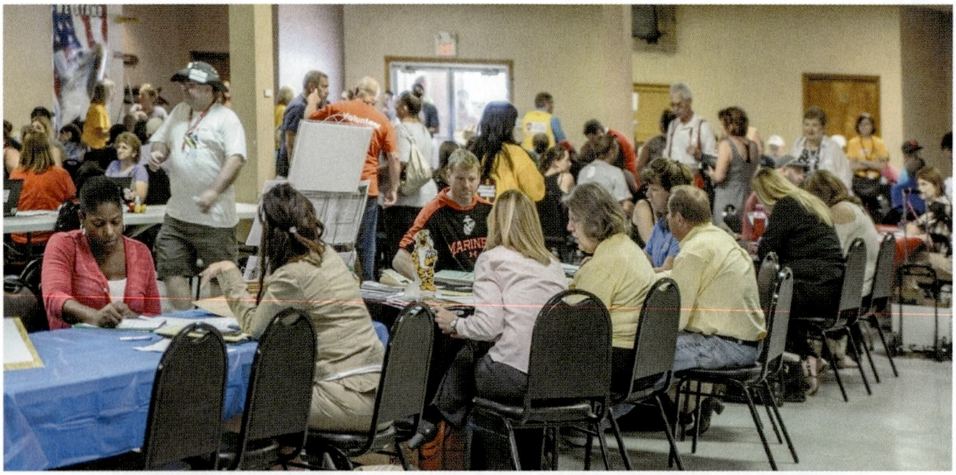

After spring 2017 floods, the Missouri EOC worked with state and local agencies and faith-based and civic volunteer organizations to set up Multi-Agency Resource Centers. These assistance centers served as one-stop shops where trained experts could help victims in many ways. They helped victims find housing, public assistance, and behavioral health counseling. They also assisted them in filling out claims forms.

be in easily accessible sites. The LEMA relies heavily on local civic and faith groups and organizations like the American Red Cross and Salvation Army to operate the PODs. The types of supplies needed are determined by the LEMA with these partners.

The local authorities or OEMs of the county or state will also set up a recovery **assistance center**. This is where victims can go to apply for financial aid and other types of recovery aid, such as help to find new housing or fill out insurance claims. Members of civic and faith groups often volunteer here. The Chamber of Commerce, Small Business Association, banks, and local businesses may also be there with assistance or special recovery loans.

County and State Assistance

As noted, if the local authorities with their community resources do not have the staff and resources to fully handle an emergency or disaster, the mayor and the LEMA or the OEM work together to seek resources from the county OEM or DOH. If the county has insufficient resources, the local authorities and county work with the state's OEM and DOH. The county and state departments are organized to follow the same NRF guidelines and ICS established by the federal government.

The governor is the incident commander of the state's responses. The key task of the state's EOC is to coordinate with the LEMA or county OEM, and with the federal agencies, if needed.

Federal Disaster Assistance

When the state does not have the resources to respond to an emergency or disaster, the governor asks the President for federal resources. FEMA then assesses whether the situation qualifies for federal aid under the Robert T. Stafford Disaster Relief and Emergency Assistance Act.

If it has been determined that federal resources are needed, a **Presidential Disaster Declaration** is issued. This permits the flow of federal money, personnel, and supplies. Yet even when federal support has been approved, states and local communities are responsible for a share of the costs.

The request for outside help can come either in anticipation of an approaching disaster or after a disaster has hit. With natural disasters, such as a hurricane, FEMA works with the state and local authorities ahead of time. FEMA can direct federal supplies and personnel to be transported in and located at a safe location as near as possible to the anticipated impact area so that so the materials can be put to use quickly.

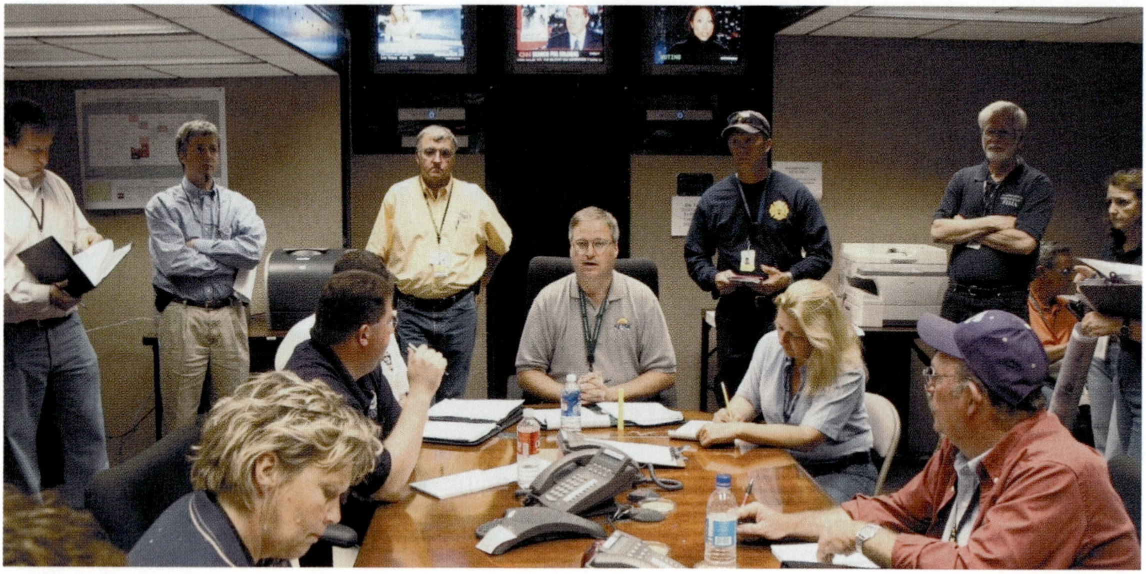

When a tornado struck Greensburg, Kansas, in May 2007, incident command briefings were held twice daily at the FEMA Emergency Operations Center that had been set up. These briefings included representatives of relief organizations and town, county, state, and federal governments.

Requested resources can include personnel, shelter, food, water, and supplies. Working with the local authorities and nonprofit partners, FEMA will establish its own EOC.

The ASPR and the CDC can also be called in to provide health-related disaster assistance, such as medical supplies, transport, equipment, laboratory services, and personnel. They will establish their own medical tents and medical supply and medication dispensing sites.

The National Disaster Medical System

When a disaster is declared and local and state medical resources are overwhelmed, the ASPR can deploy the **National Disaster Medical System (NDMS)**. The NDMS is the federal healthcare response system responsible for sending specialized medical teams, equipment, and supplies to a disaster area. The NDMS also supplies transport services and equipment to transfer ill and injured patients from disaster-stricken sites to hospitals in safe areas. If requested, the NDMS can also send medical teams to assist a hospital that is overwhelmed and in need of staff and supplies. Following Hurricane Katrina, the NDMS provided medical care teams to a hospital remaining in operation in New Orleans, since its resources were insufficient.

All members of the NDMS teams are volunteers registered in advance through a federal job site listing their state, and then they are assigned to state teams. (The registration process is covered in Chapter 6.) The volunteers participate in meetings, training sessions, and exercises with their

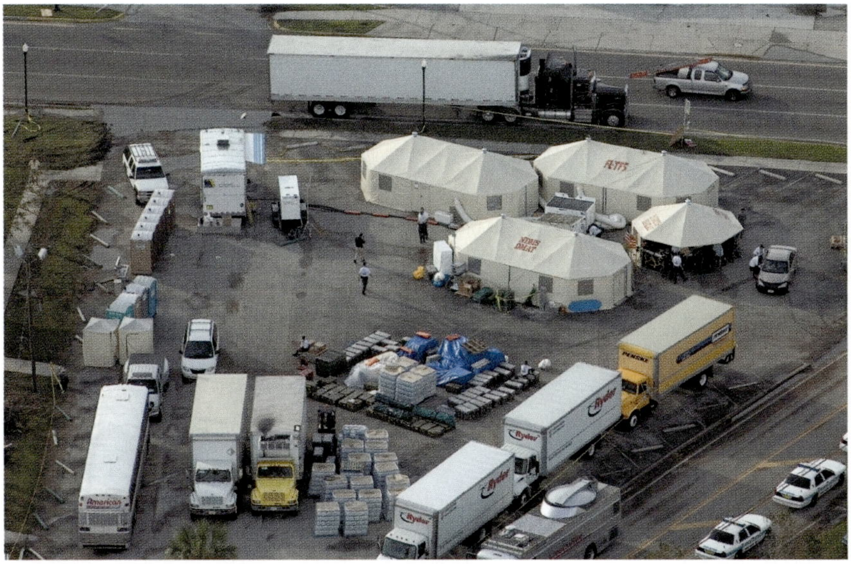

Disaster Medical Assistance Team (DMAT) tents to provide needed emergency healthcare services were set up immediately in front of a hospital in Punta Gorda, Florida, after Hurricane Charley struck on August 13, 2004.

teams on their free time. However, once deployed to a disaster site, they are officially federal employees with federal salaries and are protected by the government's malpractice and workers compensation insurance plans.

Various specialized NDMS teams that may be called in for medical assistance, including:

- **Disaster Medical Assistance Teams (DMATs)** are state or regional healthcare teams with varied healthcare professionals and paraprofiessionals. They include physicians and surgeons, EMTs and paramedics, nurses and nurse practitioners, physician assistants and respiratory therapists, and pharmacists and pharmacy technicians, among others. States or regions form their DMAT teams of healthcare professionals who live within the state so they can train together. For example, there are DMATS in Massachusetts, Texas, and Minnesota, but these teams can be sent to other states.
- **Trauma and Critical Care Teams (TCCTs)** provide surgical and critical care during disasters.
- **Disaster Mortuary Operational Response Teams (DMORTs)** are regional teams that identify victims and provide mortuary services. DMORT members include funeral directors, medical examiners, pathologists, medical records technicians, dental assistants, radiographers, behavioral health specialists (to help people whose family members have died or are missing), and support staff.

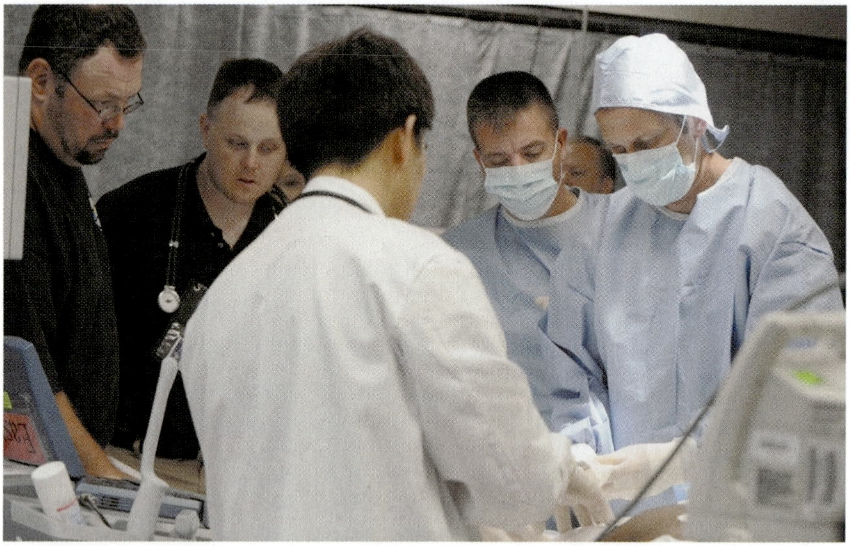

After Hurricane Ike in September 2008, members of the Iowa-1 DMAT set up mobile emergency medical tents outside of the Texas Medical Branch Hospital on Galveston Island. The hospital had a disruption of power and services. Here the team is shown treating a victim who arrived for care.

- **National Veterinary Response Teams (NVRTs)** are regional teams that provide care to search dogs and animals affected by the disaster. NVRTs include veterinarians, pathologists, animal health technicians, microbiologists, and others who assist animals who are victims and provide care to search dogs.

Assistance from the Centers for Disease Control and Prevention

During disasters, the CDC monitors the spread of diseases and provides timely and accurate health information to health departments, health care organizations, and the public.

If the local or state DOH requests additional information or guidance, the CDC provides scientific and technical training and assistance. The CDC may even send personnel to the community where the disaster occurred to provide more in-depth assistance to health departments. The CDC also helps the DOHs recover and restore public health functions after the initial response.

Government-Trained Volunteers

Government agencies can rarely handle an emergency or disaster without help from local, regional, and national volunteers. The DHS encourages and trains healthcare professionals and citizens to be volunteer responders in their own area. Sometimes they receive their training from state trainers who have been certified at the federal level, and sometimes they go to the federal training facilities themselves.

Two key types of local citizen teams are trained to assist in healthcare-related response situations.

The Medical Reserve Corps The **Medical Reserve Corps (MRC)** is a program sponsored through the ASPR for local medical professionals to be on call to help their communities in times of need. MRC units are recruited and organized through local governmental offices, faith-based groups, public health offices, hospitals, and other nongovernmental organizations. MRC volunteers train together so they are ready as a unit when a community needs additional medical resources. MRC members are not paid when they serve, and they may also be asked to help with nonemergency public health activities, such as running educational clinics on obesity reduction, healthy living, or assisting in blood or vaccination drives.

Community Emergency Response Teams Within local areas, certified volunteers may organize into teams. A **Community Emergency Response Team (CERT)** is a small group of certified volunteers organized to help in their county, city, or town with basic disaster response skills, such as fire safety, light search and rescue, disaster first aid, and medical support. CERT members receive training from federally certified CERT instructors. Once trained, CERT members can organize spontaneous volunteers at a disaster site and work with healthcare coalitions doing nonmedical tasks. These volunteers are not paid for their service or training.

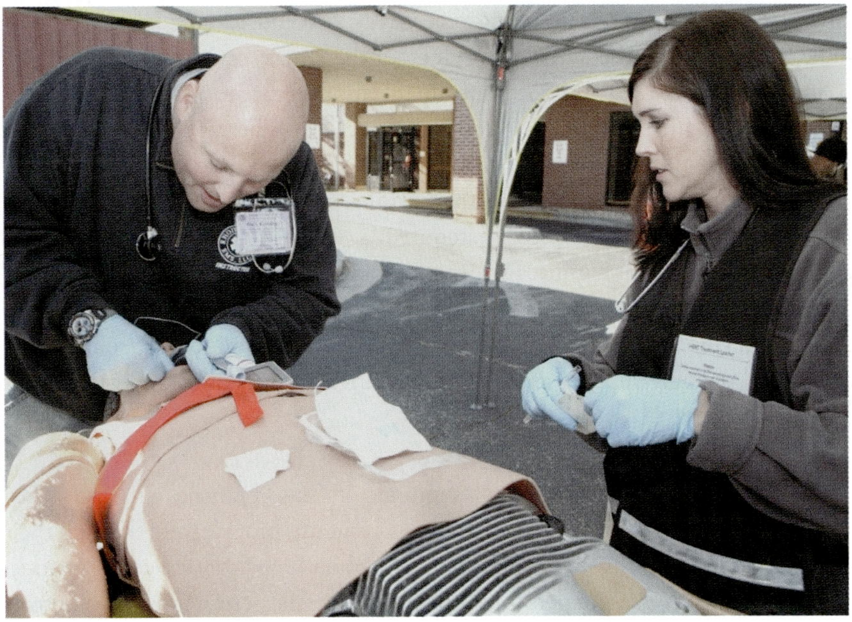

Gary Goodloff (left) from the Rhode Island Medical Reserve Corps is taking part in a Hospital Emergency Response Training for Mass Casualty Incidents course. This citizen training course is offered at the Center for Domestic Preparedness.

Civic and Religious Organizations Ready for Disasters

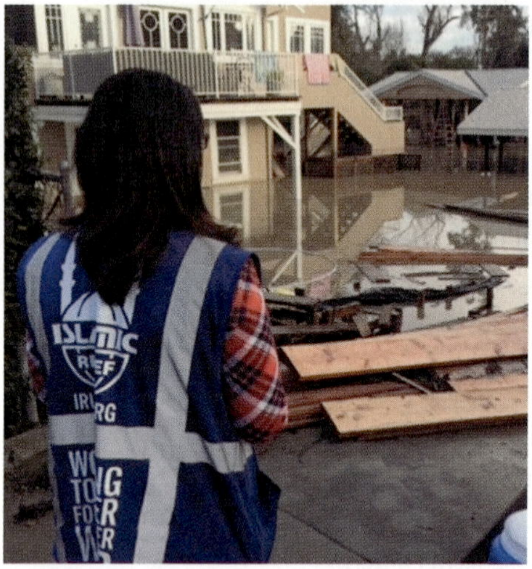

A volunteer from Islamic Relief USA worked with FEMA to distribute needed supplies and clean up after the major flooding in San Jose, California, in May 2017.

It is human nature to want to help during a disaster. Numerous civic and religious groups provide services following an emergency or disaster. Some act independently, responding to events that arise in their communities, while others collaborate in planning and response.

Over 50 community-based groups, religious organizations, and other nongovernmental organizations are members of the **National Voluntary Organizations Active in Disaster (VOAD)**. The organizations of National VOAD cooperate, communicate, and collaborate in delivering services to communities affected by disaster.

Some well-known National VOAD member groups are geared to assist in disaster response with preregistered and trained volunteers. They include the following:

American Red Cross

The American Red Cross has had a key role in emergency and disaster response in the US since 1905. After being trained, Red Cross Disaster Action Teams, run by volunteers, operate at the local level. FEMA shares responsibility with the Red Cross for planning and coordinating what are known as **mass care services**—sheltering, feeding, and providing emergency first aid to victims of disasters. The NRF delegates the tasks of carrying out these mass care services to the Red Cross, so the LEMA works with this organization to care for its citizens.

This may mean evacuating residents to places where people will be safe and where enough resources can be brought in. The Red Cross also feeds response workers and volunteers, and handles phone calls about victims from relatives who live outside the disaster area.

Also of particular significance in an emergency or disaster, the American Red Cross provides about 40% of the donated blood in the US, collected through its blood drives. This blood and other blood products are sold to hospitals and regional suppliers and are important resources during disasters.

Expand Your Knowledge

The Salvation Army USA provides a free eBook The Disaster Readiness Handbook. It includes information on how to prepare checklists of life-saving items, and forms to print out. See **http://EmDPrp2.ParadigmEducation.com/SalvationArmyUSADisasterHandbook**.

The Salvation Army

Across the country, the Salvation Army and its state branches are also a key resource. Their Emergency Disaster Services programs provide food through their mobile feeding units as well as clothing, shelter, and medical services to victims. They also feed first responders and others doing rescue. Their trained volunteers offer emotional and spiritual care to first responders and disaster victims.

Team Rubicon USA

Veterans have been trained to serve, and even after they retire, they want to continue to help their country. Team Rubicon is a nonprofit organization that "unites the skills and experiences of military veterans with first responders to rapidly deploy emergency response teams." With 40,000 registered volunteers, Team Rubicon works both domestically and internationally. Members provide the following types of services: incident management, disaster mapping and work-order management, volunteer management, debris cleanup and management, damage and impact assessment, expedient home repair, and mitigation. They also provide medical services, but only internationally, as their medical professionals can be part of DMATs or MRC teams domestically.

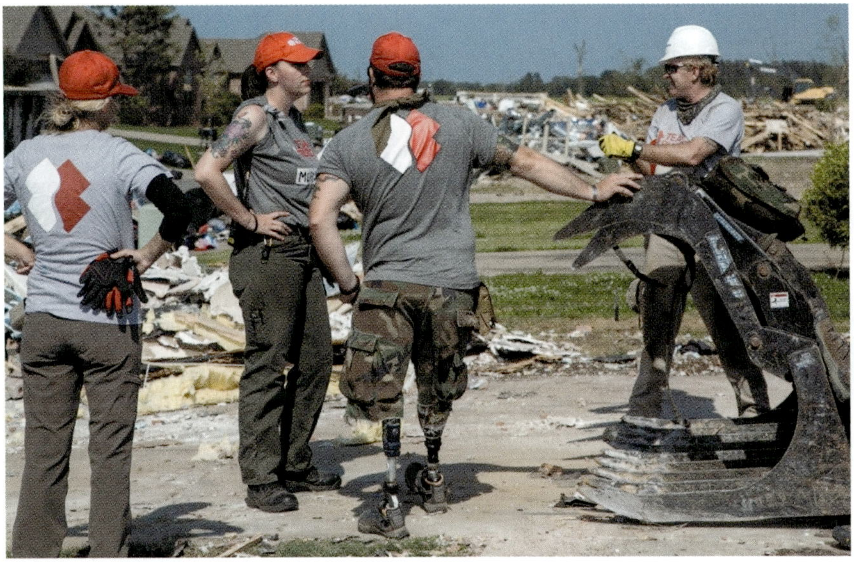

In Vilonia, Arkansas, Team Rubicon members work to clean up debris after a tornado in May 2014.

FEMA Corps

AmeriCorps NCCC (National Civilian Community Corps) partnered with FEMA to create FEMA Corps. In this program, 18-to-24 year-old citizens can serve with FEMA on a team for ten months. Older individuals train and serve as team leaders. They all gain professional skills in emergency preparedness and response. The FEMA Corps teams work on educating communities, collecting information and assessing preparedness needs, and gathering needed supplies. After a disaster, the teams are assigned with government agencies and nonprofit organizations to provide services for disaster survivors and help them completing applications for assistance. Corps members help set up shelter operations, reunite families and pets with their owners, and assess damage to public facilities, among other key tasks.

Heroes Corner

Pet Rescue

During natural disasters, many people have to evacuate without their pets and become very anxious about finding these animals. As part of the recovery efforts for Hurricane Sandy, various organizations set up Facebook pages to reunite pets with their owners, such as Pet Zealous and Hurricane Sandy Lost and Found Pets, along with Twitter accounts for the same purpose.

In New Jersey, the Governor's Office worked with the New Jersey Department of Agriculture, the US Department of Agriculture, and local chapters of The Humane Society of the United States to establish an emergency hotline and coordinate pet recovery efforts. The team worked with local responders, volunteers, and nonprofit agencies to search for, recover, care for, and reunite more than 400 pets with their owners.

Expand Your Knowledge

In 2006, Congress passed the Pets Evacuation and Transportation Standards Act (PETS Act). Local and state governments must now include pets in their emergency planning. Federal agencies can work with animal rescue and pet-oriented volunteer groups and direct disaster funds for animal welfare.

Dilemma of Unexpected Volunteers and Donations

Numerous local civic organizations and faith communities spontaneously step up to help out in any emergency or disaster. They respond in many different ways, feeding volunteers or victims, offering emotional counseling, finding lost pets or taking care of abandoned animals, or helping in cleanup.

Many people will send donations or just show up at the scene to try to rescue survivors or pitch in. They are of great assistance, but unfortunately this outpouring of help can also cause additional problems if not carefully coordinated through a group or the local authorities.

As an example, thousands of mutual aid responders and volunteers poured into Joplin, Missouri immediately after a tornado in 2011. The extra workers helped Joplin respond to the massive destruction and cleanup, but they also presented challenges for those managing the incident. These volunteers were not part of the organized response and their actions were not coordinated activities. Finding housing and food for them was difficult. They also needed to be put to work in the right places so that they didn't get in the way of other work being done. That is why it is important to preregister to volunteer or connect with a group that is part of the response effort.

Throughout all the four stages of emergency and disaster response, the local authorities are the leaders. Yet a successful efficient response depends on all partners in the community and in the state and federal governments doing their jobs well. All healthcare professionals need to understand how emergency and disaster response works to know their roles in it.

Chapter Summary

The US has an organized system of emergency and disaster preparedness built on the principles of comprehensive emergency management and its four phases: prevention and mitigation of risks, preparedness and training, response, and recovery. The National Response Framework provides the guidance for planning and management, whereas the National Incident Management System provides the Incident Command System template for organizing a response to emergencies and disasters.

All levels of government (local, tribal, county, state, and federal) plan for disasters and organize their response based on the federal guidance. The local authorities always lead the response management. Citizen volunteer groups and nongovernmental organizations also play key roles in disaster response.

Additional Resources

To extend the content presented in this chapter, take advantage of the resources available through the chapter's eBook resource links and the end-of-chapter links. These resources include informational supplements and flash cards for terms and abbreviations.

Key Terms	
assets	mutual aid
assistance center	Point of Distribution
comprehensive emergency management	preparedness
emergency operations center	Presidential Disaster Declaration
emergency exercises	recovery
incident commander	response
incident command center	scalable
mass care services	Threat and Hazard Identification and Risk Assessment
mitigation	unified command

Recognizing Terms

Choose the word or phrase from the list of key terms that best matches each of the following descriptions. Your instructor may ask you to submit your work for grading or may provide you with an answer key for self-assessment.

1. Establishes ways that communities will assist each other in responding to or recovering from a disaster ________
2. Needed to receive federal assistance for disaster response ________
3. What communities and states do to prevent or minimize any emergencies that could occur from hazards ________
4. Services for victims, such as sheltering, feeding, and providing health services and Psychological First Aid ________
5. A place for victims to go to access resources and get aid after a disaster ________
6. The personnel, equipment, and other supplies that are provided during a response to an emergency ________
7. A four-phase approach to planning for and responding to disasters ________
8. When all agencies with responsibilities for handling an incident work together to establish and implement a single, coordinated plan ________
9. The phase of emergency management where a community gets everything ready for activation if a disaster occurs ________
10. The actions taken before, during, or immediately after the emergency incident ________

Reviewing Concepts

Choose the response that best answers the question or completes the sentence. Your instructor may ask you to submit your work for grading or may provide you with an answer key for self-assessment.

1. Which phase of comprehensive emergency management involves creating evacuation plans?
   a. mitigation
   b. preparedness
   c. response
   d. recovery

2. What is one of the initial tasks for first responders in an emergency?
   a. setting up the incident command structure on site
   b. seeking assistance from the federal government
   c. assessing the cost of damages
   d. determining what has happened
3. Who must originate a request for federal disaster relief?
   a. congressional representative
   b. governor of a state
   c. head of FEMA
   d. head of a LEMA
4. Which is not one of the four steps involved in disaster planning?
   a. identifying your capabilities
   b. organizing key personnel, equipment, and supplies
   c. conducting drills to test the plans
   d. requesting federal assistance
   e. arranging for mutual aid
5. Which team belonging to the National Disaster Medical System provides victim identification services?
   a. Disaster Medical Assistance Team
   b. Disaster Mortuary Operational Response Team
   c. National Pharmacy Response Team
   d. Federal Emergency Management Team
6. Why is an incident command system (ICS) important in disaster response?
   a. Many agencies need to organize themselves differently according to the type of disaster.
   b. The LEMA needs someone to go out to the site of a disaster.
   c. ICS makes clear whom everyone reports to and whose orders they must follow.
   d. The federal government needs to be able to command an incident.
7. Which federal agencies provide direction for emergency preparedness?
   a. FEMA, FDA, CDC, DOT
   b. DHS, FEMA, EPA, DOD
   c. DOE, DOJ, DOS, FEMA
   d. FEMA, DHS, ASPR, CDC

8. How do nongovernmental organizations work with LEMAs and FEMA in disasters?
   a. Help unite pets with their owners.
   b. Plan and coordinate what are known as mass care services.
   c. Help transport victims to safe evacuation sites.
   d. Help with cleanup of debris.
   e. All of these answers are correct.

9. Who is responsible for managing a response?
   a. the local officials
   b. the county officials
   c. the state officials
   d. the federal agencies

10. What is National Voluntary Organizations Active in Disaster?
    a. a national organization with chapters to collect donations for emergencies
    b. a national response organization with local chapters to organize volunteers
    c. a network of organizations that cooperate, communicate, coordinate, and collaborate in delivering services to communities affected by disaster
    d. a federal agency that organizes volunteers after disaster

11. Whole community preparedness is
    a. being sure that everyone knows everyone in the community.
    b. including children in planning for disasters.
    c. working with everyone to protect people of all neighborhoods and ages.
    d. having a translator at every planning meeting.

12. What are ways that you can expand your knowledge about preparedness?
    a. training and drills at work
    b. continuing education courses offered by professional organizations and schools
    c. courses on the Internet and in your local healthcare facility and community
    d. All of these answers are correct.

13. What occurs when volunteers show up at the scene of disaster without being registered?
    a. They may expect to be provided a place to stay.
    b. They may get in the way because they are not coordinated properly.
    c. There may not be enough protective equipment for them to help.
    d. They may help clean up the debris.
14. Why did many people lose pets during Hurricane Sandy?
    a. The pets couldn't swim.
    b. The pets could not go to the evacuation centers.
    c. The pets ran out of food and water.
    d. The pets caught a cold from being wet.

Exploring Emergency Preparedness Issues

Complete the following activities to further explore the concepts found in this chapter. Your instructor may ask you to submit your work for grading or may provide you with guidance for self-assessment.

1. Go to www.fema.gov//disasters. This FEMA page lists the latest Federal (Presidential) Disaster Declarations. There you can search for the disasters that occurred in your state. Summarize this information in a one-page report.
2. Contact the LEMA in your community. What types of emergencies are they planning for? Are they planning for more than one kind of disaster, or are they using an all-hazards approach? Does their plan include healthcare facilities where you work or might work? How are they included? Discuss your responses to these questions in one or two pages.
3. Contact a local hospital and ask how to volunteer to role-play as a victim in a drill. If time allows and you are able to volunteer, write a two-page report about your observations and the types of activities your profession carried out in the drill. If you noticed that the exercise identified a weakness in the response, include that in your report (as well as your recommendation for improving the emergency response).

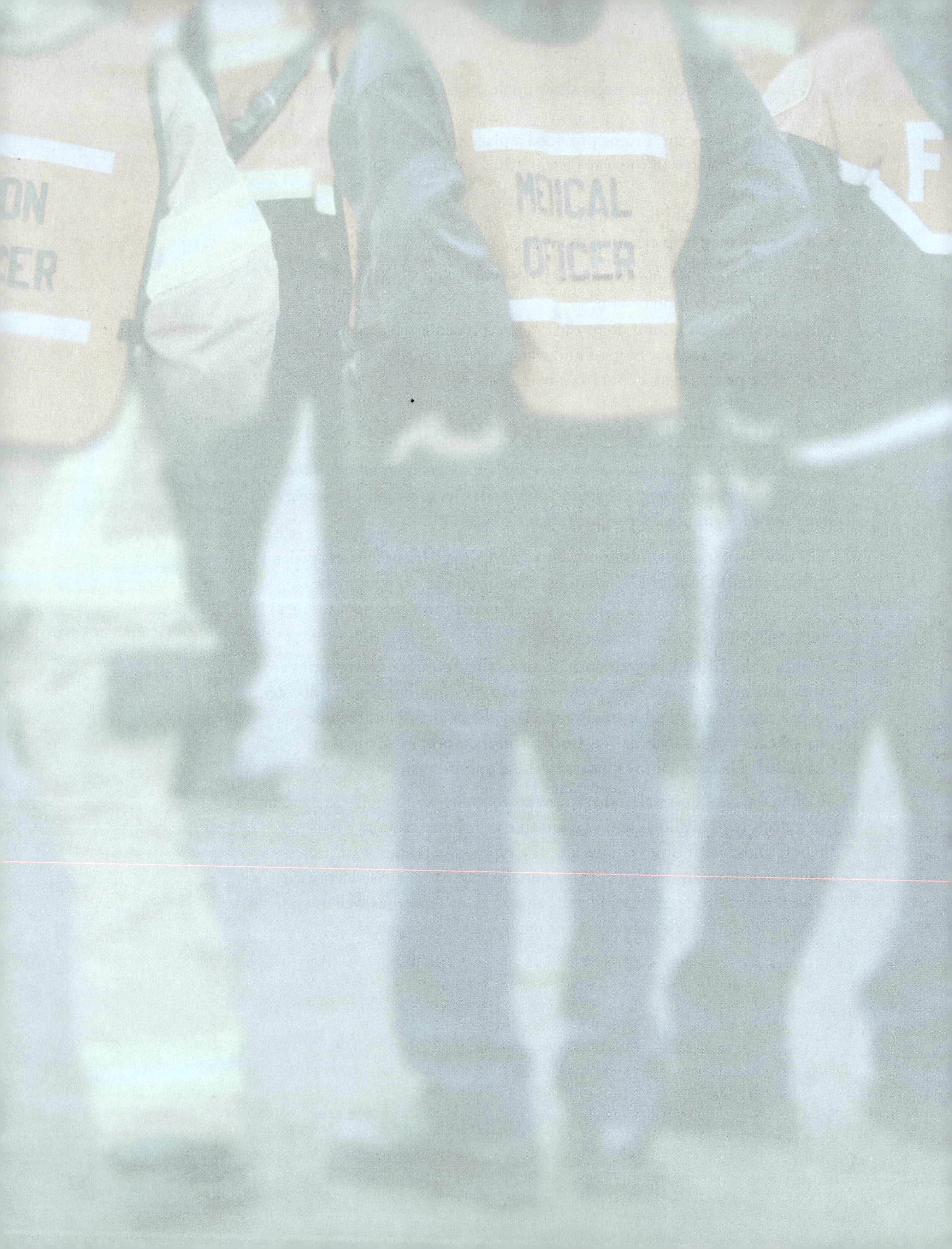

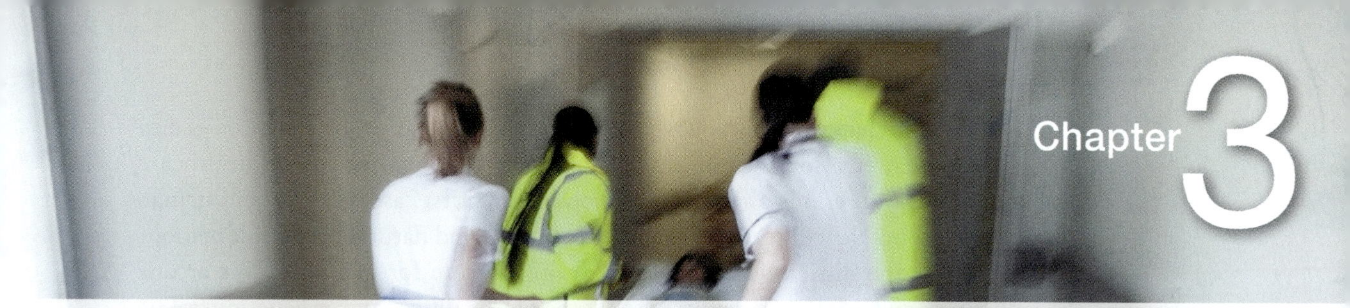

Chapter 3

Healthcare Planning, Challenges, and Case Studies

What You Will Learn

- How hospitals and other healthcare facilities prepare for emergencies and disasters
- The unique challenges hospital and other healthcare facilities plan for
- What is included in a hospital evacuation plan
- How emergency and disaster managers and health professionals responded to different types of hazards in past incidents
- What strategies and actions have worked well
- What problems could be prevented through preparedness and different approaches

Each emergency and disaster is unique, with different causes, situations, health effects, patient outcomes, and available resources. Every healthcare facility must look at the most likely risks it may face, and how its staff and resources would address them. Hospitals and other healthcare facilities need to create emergency plans. To do so, they consider what other facilities and healthcare personnel have encountered in past disasters to help develop strategies for handling future disasters more effectively and efficiently.

This chapter explores how healthcare systems plan and what they need to consider. It also looks at three significant disasters where the healthcare system was seriously affected or involved. The first case, Hurricane Katrina's effects on New Orleans, is about a weather-related natural disaster. It demonstrates the difficulties involved in trying to care for many patients at one time, and deal with power loss, damaged facilities, and evacuations. The second case study, the Boston Marathon bombings, describes the healthcare system's response to a terrorist bombing. The third case describes how a state laboratory, local hospital, and public health system responded to the first US case of a highly infectious disease—the Ebola Virus Disease.

Key Acronyms	
CT	computed tomography
DOD	US Department of Defense
DSHS	Department of State Health Services
ED	emergency department
EVD	Ebola Virus Disease
FAST	focused assessment with sonography for trauma
FDA	US Food and Drug Administration
HICS	Hospital Incident Command System
LRN	Laboratory Response Network
PPE	personal protective equipment

Healthcare Facility Preparedness

The Joint Commission on Accreditation of Health Organizations, known as **The Joint Commission**, is the national organization for certifying hospitals, long-term care facilities, behavioral health facilities, and ambulatory care clinics. To receive accreditation, these facilities must develop and communicate to staff detailed emergency operations plans that work for any type of emergency or disaster.

Federal agencies also have requirements for emergency preparedness for healthcare facilities. Hospitals and health clinics that serve Medicare patients and receive federal money must follow federal guidelines on preparedness, such as the Emergency Preparedness Rule discussed in Chapter 1.

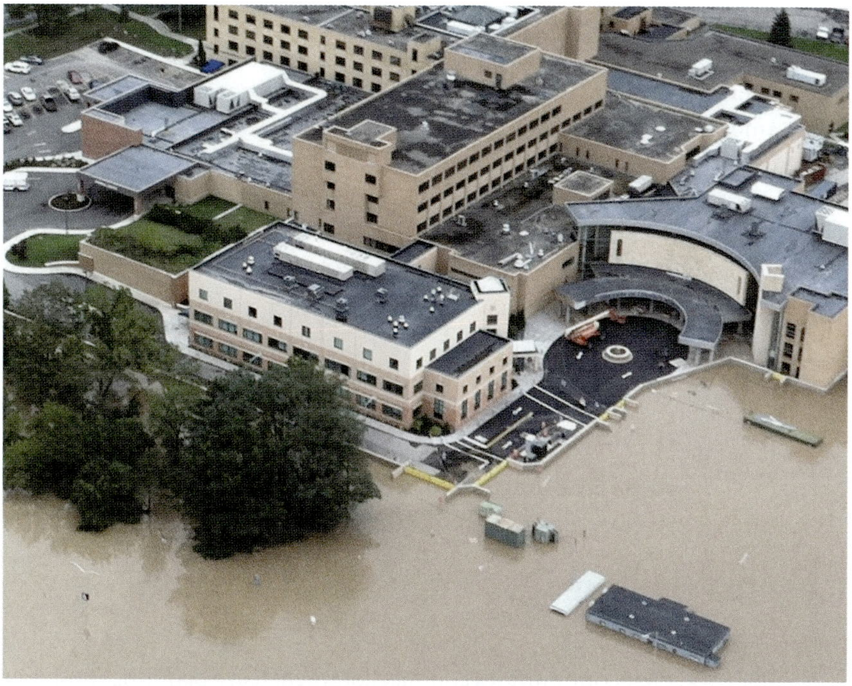

To protect Our Lady of Lourdes Hospital in Binghamton, New York, flood walls were built with hazard mitigation funds from FEMA and New York State after damage in 2006. These walls proved key for preventing damage during Tropical Storm Lee in September 2011, though waters from the Susquehanna River covered the parking lots.

Federal Healthcare Response Framework and Resources

To help healthcare facilities and departments of health within all communities prepare, the Assistant Secretary for Preparedness and Response (ASPR) provides guidance, standards, resources, and assistance. As explained in Chapter 2, the ASPR is the national leader in supporting health and medical services during emergencies and disasters. The office coordinates the federal health and medical response and works with other federal agencies and with state and local governments to strengthen their preparedness and response.

Developing Healthcare Capabilities

The ASPR developed guidelines for healthcare coalitions (HCCs), including hospitals and Emergency Medical Services (EMS), to be ready for emergencies and disasters. *The 2017–2022 Health Care Preparedness and Response*

Capabilities describes the four capabilities, or skills and resources, in these areas:

- **Healthcare and medical readiness:** Comprehensive preparation among the HCC members by identifying hazards and risks, developing strong relationships, and coordinating the planning, training, exercising, and managing of resources
- **Healthcare and medical response coordination:** Integration of the preparedness of each healthcare organization into the HCC system in a coordinated way by sharing information, managing processes, and resources
- **Continuity of healthcare delivery:** Provisions for the continuity of healthcare services with well trained, well-educated, well-equipped personnel
- **Medical surge readiness:** Accommodations to ensure that the healthcare system can deliver medical care to many more people than usual

Hospital Emergency Operations Planning Challenges

In the same way that communities conduct comprehensive planning, hospitals develop a hospital emergency operations plan (EOP). The EOP is designed to ensure the facility's ability to provide quality patient care during a disaster. Both The Joint Commission and federal guidelines require hospitals to follow a **Hospital Incident Command System (HICS)**. The EOP assigns the HICS command and staff responsibilities on **job action sheets**. The incident commander is usually the healthcare facility's chief executive or chief operating officer. The location of the command center—the emergency operations center—within the healthcare facility is determined as part of the EOP.

Once the EOP and HICS are activated, the hospital can work efficiently with other agencies responding to an emergency or disaster because they all are using the same terminology and organizing principles.

In addition to establishing the roles and command center for the HICS, the EOP identifies and makes plans to address the following:

- How, when, and by whom the emergency and disaster response should be activated
- How staff members will be notified when they are needed
- How staff assignments will be made
- How staff and patients will be kept safe from harm
- Procedures for providing patient care
- Proper inventory levels of supplies, medications, and equipment to maintain patient care

Expand Your Knowledge

As noted in Chapter 1, healthcare facilities must adhere to the Emergency Preparedness Rule to receive Medicare and Medicaid reimbursement. For the requirements, visit **http://EmDPrp2.ParadigmEducation.com/Medicare-Medicaid**.

Web

- Roles of support and security staff
- Procedures for communicating with the Local Emergency Management Agency (LEMA) and other HCC members
- How communication with the media is to be handled
- Agreements with other healthcare facilities in the HCC for mutual aid and support
- Criteria and plans for evacuating the building and establishing care at an alternative site
- Provisions for testing the EOP through training exercises

In addition to these elements, a hospital and other health facilities must consider the many common challenges that arise during disasters.

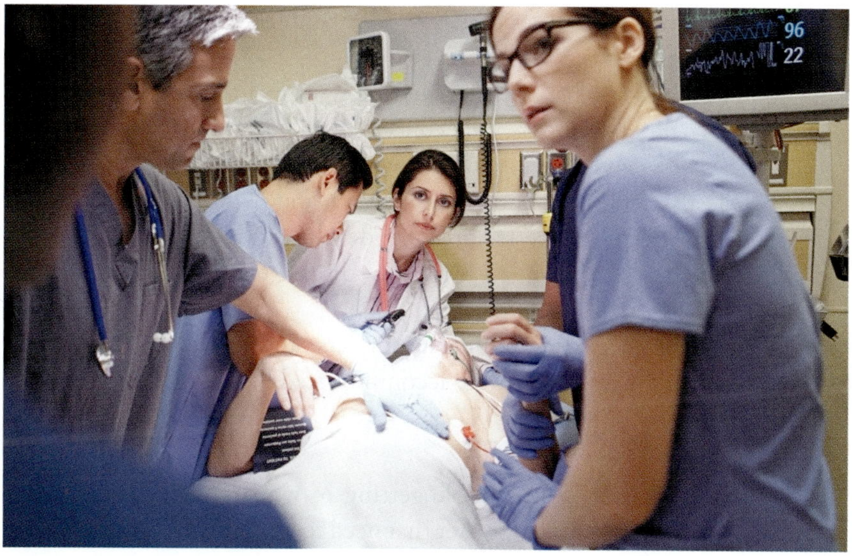

Hospitals have to make Emergency Operations Plans to be ready for a rush of many patients needing triage, diagnostic tests, and treatments even if the hospital may itself have sustained damage or power outages.

Medical Surge

During an emergency or disaster, many people might need medical attention simultaneously. A sudden increase in the number of patients at the same time is a **medical surge** (also known as a "patient surge"). The following events can occur:

- An insufficient number of ambulances and EMTs may be available for the large number of patients requiring help.
- A large volume of victims may begin arriving on their own soon after an incident. The facility may not be prepared to receive or treat them

and may need to reassign staff from other units to the emergency department (ED) or call in staff on their days off.

- Some victims may go to the nearest facility, even if it cannot handle the type of injury or the number of patients that need medical attention. Others with less severe injuries or non-life-threatening illness may go home to visit the doctors or hospitals where they usually seek medical care.
- Victims may be of varied ages and not be from the area where the incident occurs. They may speak different languages, and interpreters may not be available.
- Children may be separated from their parents.
- Testing and lab facilities may be overwhelmed, and labs may need to send samples to another lab. They need a preexisting agreement to do so in a timely way.
- Some people who have not have been physically injured or ill may come to the facility because they are concerned about what has just happened to them or people they know, or what might happen to them. These people also require response, observation, and perhaps care.
- Patients already in the facility may develop additional complications from the stress or from an infectious disease or a type of contamination if it is part of the incident.
- Family members, community responders, and the media may swarm to the facility and need to be accommodated.

Additional Staff Issues

Not only may the staff have trouble getting to work, other staffing issues occur during an emergency or disaster that need to be considered for planning. They include:

- Staff may have to work longer hours than normal and work a different schedule.
- Certain kinds of health professionals may be in short supply to meet the increased demands. For example, healthcare facilities may need more health professionals to handle increased lab work or X-rays and other imaging. This is where mutual aid agreements with other health facilities are key in planning.
- Staff may not be working with their usual coworkers. Professionals from other facilities may be given emergency privileges to assist in different specialized areas or provide clinical care and are not likely to be familiar with the exact procedures or resources of the facility.

- To have sufficient staff to handle a disaster's medical surge, elective procedures are likely to be cancelled. However, people with chronic illnesses or special medical needs will still require ongoing care, such as pregnant women who go into labor and people who have asthma attacks, heart attacks, strokes, and accidents. Meeting these needs requires planning and coordination.

Healthcare coalitions support each other by providing staff for overwhelmed hospitals during a medical surge. With a large-scale incident, the hospital administrators may grant disaster privileges to local volunteers licensed as independent practitioners (to assist the hospital staff), and the state may send in state medical response teams. Another staffing resource for disasters is the Medical Reserve Corps. If a presidential disaster has been declared, the ASPR may send in Disaster Medical Assistance Teams (DMATs).

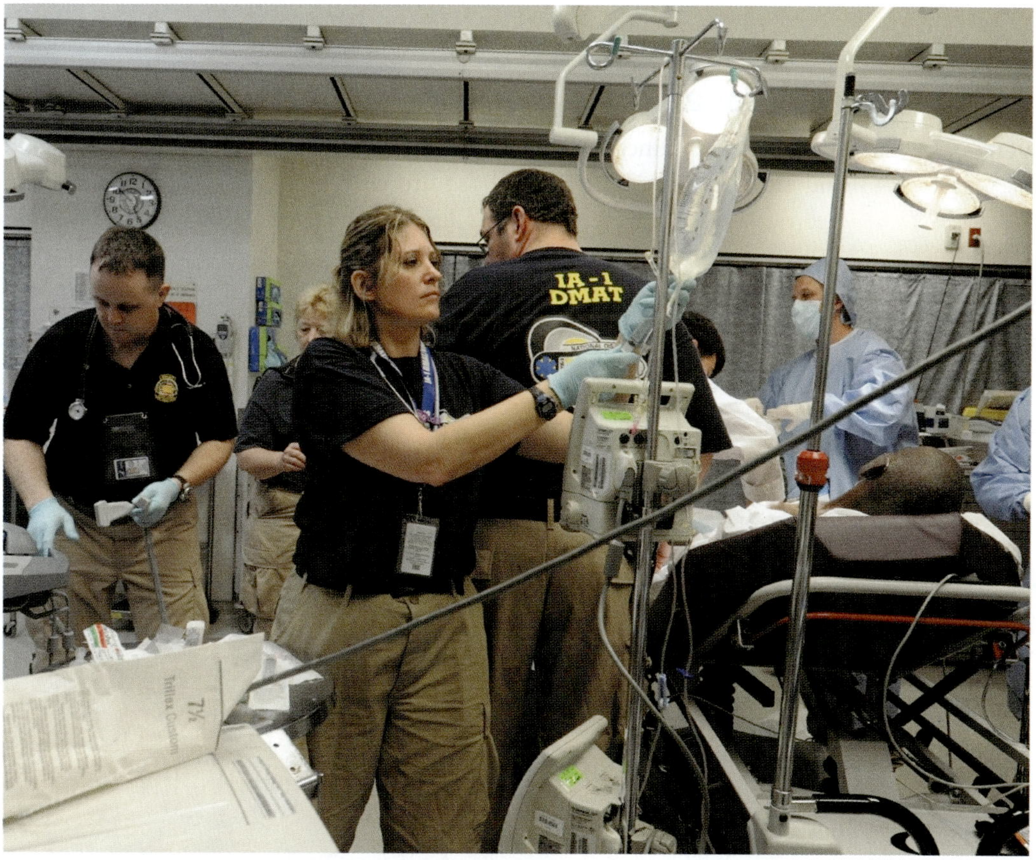

After Hurricane Ike, the Iowa-1 DMAT set up at the University of Texas Medical Branch to assist with patients on Galveston Island, Texas, in September 2008.

Communications Issues

Expand Your Knowledge

Hospitals have to make plans for how to use social media tools. See the digital supplement, "Social Media Tools for Emergency Communication."

Cell phone and telephone lists, email blasts, and text messages are common ways to notify all staff quickly. In a disaster, though, phone and electrical lines often go down. Cell phone connections become jammed and the Internet networks crash. It may be difficult to communicate with colleagues within the healthcare facility as well as with others outside, making it hard to contact staff who are on-call, receive disaster updates or lab results, or report lab results. Healthcare facilities need to establish plans to handle these potential issues.

The emergency operation plan should have a contact number outside the region so, if necessary, employees can check it if cellular connections and telephone lines are not working. If hospitals and other healthcare facilities have some power and Internet access, they can also communicate crucial information with their established social media tools, such as their public and staff web pages, Facebook, and Twitter.

Additional Power Outage Problems

Be Aware

After a storm, power outages may persist for days or weeks, and the heat or cold can do great harm. In 2017, eight residents in a Florida nursing home died from heat exposure after Hurricane Irma. The backup generators and portable air conditioning units were not able to adequately cool the entire facility.

Radiology machines, various monitoring devices, life support equipment, and sterilization equipment all require electricity, as do elevators. When electrical lines are down, facilities also may not have enough power to light hallways and rooms. Although most hospitals have generators and plan to have fuel on hand, they may not have enough to keep the generators running if the power outage lasts a long time. They should maintain a stock of fuel supplies to keep the generators running for numerous days.

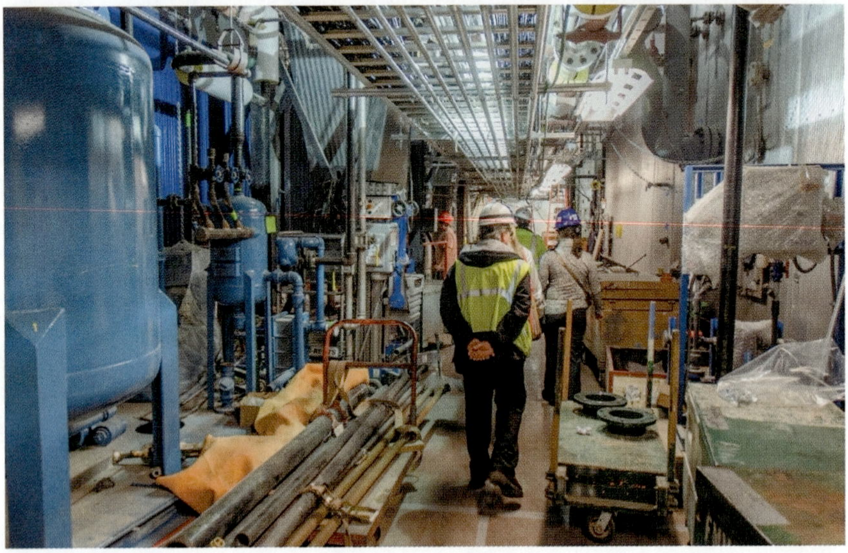

Two years after Hurricane Sandy, work goes on to build a dual-fuel power generating system to protect NYU Langone Medical Center from future power outages.

A Closer Look

Maintaining Vaccines and Medications

Some vaccines and medications must always be kept refrigerated or frozen. If you are responsible for them during a power outage, use the following guidelines:

- Do not unplug the power cord of refrigerators or freezers, because the unit will resume operating as soon as power is restored.
- Do not open freezers and refrigerators until power is restored.
- Do not transfer vaccines or medications from the refrigerator to the unpowered freezer. If the power is restored and they freeze, they may not be usable.
- If you have a secure unit with a reliable power source, transfer any vaccine and medication to that unit.
- As soon as power is restored, record the temperature in both the refrigerator and the freezer. Also, record the duration of the outage.
- Do not discard the vaccines and medications. Separate questionable stock from new stock. Store the questionable units in containers that are marked, stapled, and banded until their efficacy can be determined.
- If you are concerned about the efficacy of any such stock, do not administer it until you have consulted with the state or local health department or the manufacturer.

Power to maintain constant refrigeration must be planned for. Receiving medications from sources outside of the hospital requires setting up the proper storage conditions for them. Of special concern are medicines and vaccines that require refrigeration at a constant temperature. It is important for laboratory and pharmacy personnel to know the types of products that will be damaged by lack of refrigeration, such as laboratory testing supplies, medications, and solutions used in intravenous therapy.

Be Aware

Older facilities may have battery-operated temperature monitors. Staff must read and record the temperatures each shift. However, new refrigerator units have built-in monitoring systems. If these go down with the power, other temperature monitoring devices must be used.

Loss of Healthcare Records

Patient medical records contain crucial information that guides diagnosis and treatment. Pharmacists, pharmacy technicians, and providers depend on medication records. They house information on the drugs and dosages a patient is taking and any drug interactions, allergic reactions, or drug allergies to avoid dangerous drug reactions.

Yet in emergencies and disasters, access to these records can be wiped out or hampered. Most healthcare facilities and pharmacies use only electronic medical records, and these records may not be available if power is out or computers or storage sites are damaged.

Be Aware

Pharmacies hit by disasters can also lose access to their records. Independent pharmacies must plan for this possibility. Most chain pharmacies share records of prescriptions filled and patient profiles with each other, which provides additional protection.

Hospitals and other healthcare facilities need to protect their records through remote backup systems that are stored in another physical location. For instance, some hospital systems in New York City use backup systems located across the Hudson River in New Jersey. Most large healthcare facilities have backup systems running incrementally throughout the day. Smaller medical offices and pharmacies should back up at least daily to an external hard drive for additional protection and perhaps a remote online location. Servers also should have a built-in slow shutdown to avoid data loss in case of a sudden power outage. Implementing such systems is an important role in emergency and disaster preparedness.

Hospitals and healthcare facilities, clinics, and pharmacies often use different software systems that organize their medical records differently. Because of this, they cannot always communicate with each other. When patients are evacuated to other facilities, continuity of healthcare is threatened if the patients aren't accompanied by written records of their conditions, treatments, medications, and dosages. During a disaster, hospitals and long-term care facilities may need to create a one-page summary on paper to send with the patient if he or she is transferred to another facility.

Facility Evacuation Plans

All EOPs describe the facility's evacuation plans. **Evacuation** is the organized, phased, and supervised withdrawal of people from a dangerous or potentially dangerous area. Examples of when an evacuation of a medical facility may be necessary include an earthquake, fire, flood, hurricane, or utility failure. Evacuation plans include procedures for moving patients from their rooms to an area where they gather and are prepared to be transported, called a **staging area**, where they can be moved on gurneys or in wheelchairs to a vehicle for transport.

Evacuations require everyone in the facility—patients, visitors, staff—to be moved out of the building and transported to a new location. An evacuation can take 36 to 72 hours and is labor-intensive. Staff members must notify patients' families and prepare and move patients. Facilities can reach out to key staff members who are not on duty to come in to assist in the process when needed.

Deciding to Evacuate

Evacuating a health facility is so challenging that the risks have to be carefully weighed. If the danger does not seem pressing, facilities often take a wait-and-see approach, determining that it is best to wait until they have more information. Authorities may decide that it is safer to shelter-in-place,

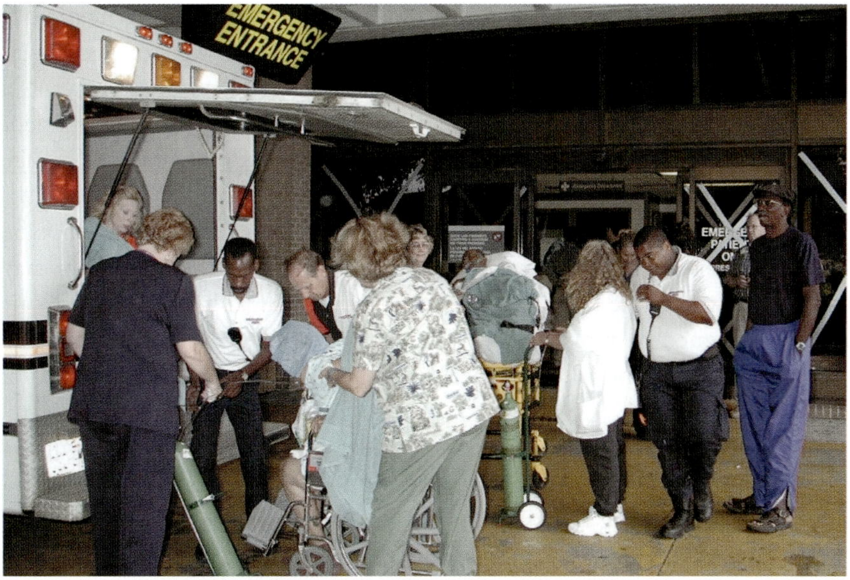

In preparation for Hurricane Lili, staff members at Christus St. Mary's Hospital in Port Arthur, Texas, evacuate their patients to other hospitals outside the hurricane evacuation zone.

or stay in a safe place in the building, especially if local roads are not passable. If a decision is made to shelter in place, patients and staff remain where they are or are moved to the most secure area of the facility.

When deciding whether to evacuate a facility, the healthcare administrators and staff should consider:

- The condition and physical limitations of each patient
- Whether a patient needs a ventilator or respiratory support during transport
- The capacity of the receiving facilities to take care of the sickest patients
- The distance to the receiving facility
- The number of and patient capacity of the evacuation staging areas for transport
- The time and staff needed for moving patients and the desired timeline to move to the staging areas and then onto transport
- The resources available for transport, such as vans, buses, helicopters, and semitrailers. Facilities often have contracts with transportation providers for potential evacuations.

Evacuation plans include **memorandums of understanding** with other facilities, which are agreements to receive patients in case of evacuation. The facility's EOP will include an assignment of job tasks, including during an evacuation. For instance, certain staff members may be assigned to turning off or securing medical gases, equipment, medications, lab specimens, or medical records.

Moving Patients If a facility is evacuated, you may be asked to help move patients to the staging area. Many patients will be able to walk on their own. Those who cannot will need to be evacuated by wheelchair or stretcher. If a patient has his or her own wheelchair, it is important to transport the patient together with the chair, since many of these chairs are customized. (If they need to be separated, they should be reunited as soon as possible.)

In some incidents, such as fires and earthquakes, elevators cannot be used, and patients must be carried down or up the stairs. A relay team may be needed with more than three flights. Some medical facilities have "stair chairs" designed to move people up or down stairs. However, patients in wheelchairs would need to be wheeled to the stairs and transferred one at a time to a stair chair.

Special attention is also required for patients with visual or hearing impairments. The visually impaired patients will need leading by the elbow, and those who are hearing impaired may need written instructions. Interpreters will be needed for non-English-speaking patients.

The evacuation plan must include a process of accounting for all staff members and patients before, during, and after an evacuation. This is critical because knowing that everyone is out and accounted for can prevent unnecessary, time-consuming, and potentially dangerous search and rescue operations.

A Closer Look

Know the Evacuation Plan

Healthcare facilities need to train employees in evacuation procedures. Each evacuation plan contains the following:

- Actions to take in the event of an alarm or order to evacuate immediately
- Nearest exits and an alternative route
- A designated staff person in your department responsible for taking attendance
- Your responsibilities for moving patients
- Special responsibility assignments, such as shutting down critical operations or protecting equipment
- Location of staging areas inside and outside the building and the one you are assigned to
- How to check in after a community evacuation. Many employers ask employees to check in through the Internet and to provide contact information.

Learn the evacuation procedures for your facility so that you can help keep yourself and others safe.

To account for each patient, health professionals need to complete a tracking form (electronic or paper if power/computers are out) that includes:

- Medical record number or patient identifier
- Time the patient left facility
- Name of transporting agency
- Medical record summary sent with patient (yes or no)
- Medications sent with patient (yes or no)
- Family notified of transfer (yes or no). Who?

Damage to a Healthcare Facility

A hospital also needs to plan for how to respond if the facility has itself been impaired before the patients could be evacuated. Some of the common damages to facilities that occur are the following:

- The building may be partially or completely destroyed. It may continue to operate or be so badly damaged it needs to be evacuated and closed.
- Besides power and communications systems, the facility may be cut off from its water supply and waste disposal.
- If certain chemicals, drugs, heavy equipment, and radiation devices are damaged or overturned, they can become hazardous, jeopardizing the health of staff and patients.
- In a disaster that lasts a long time, healthcare facilities may become isolated and run out of food and essential supplies, such as pharmaceuticals, splints, bandages, and blood.
- Healthcare facilities can also run out of the necessary equipment and the parts to keep them running when many more patients require care in a short time span.

Healthcare facilities need to consider these contingencies when developing their EOPs.

Heroes Corner

Tornado Tragedies and Rescue

A 2011 tornado caused catastrophic damage to the St. John's Regional Medical Center and other healthcare facilities in Joplin, Missouri. Although many patients and staff died, the medical staff who survived transferred the hospitalized patients to the parking lot. They assessed over 1,100 injured there. Volunteers used pickup trucks, ambulances, and other undamaged vehicles to help the medical personnel transfer critical patients to Freeman Health System, one mile away, and to St. John's Hospital in Springfield, Missouri. Within 90 minutes after the tornado struck, St. John's personnel had evacuated 183 patients from the destroyed facility.

Emergency Operations Plan Drills

To ensure preparedness, The Joint Commission requires hospitals to practice their emergency operation plans twice a year. These tests can be either activated in response to an actual incident or conducted as a planned exercise. They should be designed to determine the level of effectiveness of the HICS communication and coordination systems within the hospital.

Additionally, if hospitals have an emergency department, at least one of the annual exercises must include volunteers who role-play as patients to provide the sense of a medical surge.

It is essential that every healthcare worker be familiar with the following:

- The codes used by the facility to signal that there is an emergency. For example, a facility might use the ringing of four alarms or bells, or announce an "amber code" to signal an emergency.
- What the facility plan expects of each department
- Whom workers report to and the chain of command
- His or her own professional responsibilities during an emergency or disaster
- How supervisors will notify staff not currently within the facility that the plan is activated

If you are notified of an incident while on duty, go to your assigned location as soon as possible. You may be asked to remain in this position or be reassigned. If you are notified of an incident when you are at home, check any contact phone numbers or social media channels. If there are no specific messages, report to work at your usual shift. Do not stay at home waiting for directions.

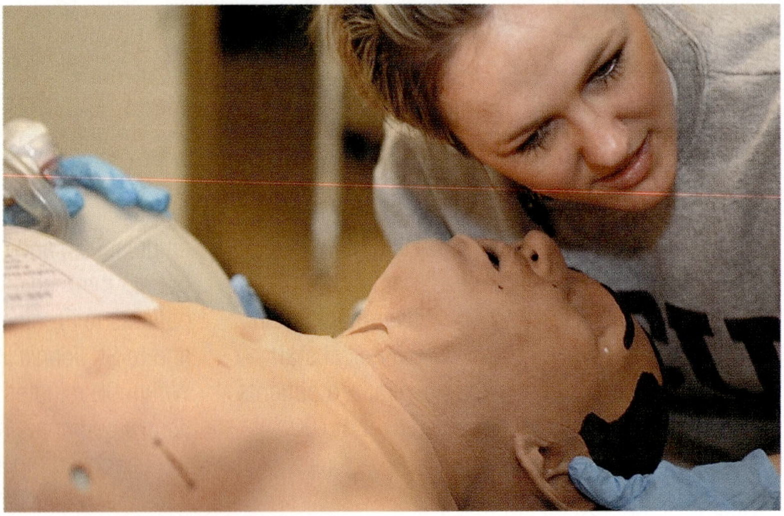

In a mass casualty simulation drill, Michelle Hollingsworth, a registered nurse, listens for breathing during the Hospital Emergency Response Training (HERT) for Mass Casualty Incidents course at the Center for Domestic Preparedness.

Preparation at Medical Clinics and Offices

In addition to hospitals, it is important for all healthcare facilities, including long-term care, behavioral healthcare, and ambulatory care clinics and medical offices, to remain open during emergencies and disasters if they are not in an evacuation area. If a facility is part of a larger healthcare system, some staff members may be reassigned to a site where they are needed more urgently.

The healthcare providers who work outside of hospitals play a major role in ensuring continuity of care during a disaster, serving the chronic disease patients and others in need of medical care. Patients with illnesses, such as those needing dialysis or with asthma, will get sicker if they do not receive needed medical treatment.

Clinics and offices as well as pharmacies are required to have their own emergency plans. The office manager often creates the plan. The EOPs need a contingency plan for backup power, staff notification, communications, patient records, refrigeration, and other issues. The EOP should also contain procedures for evacuating the building, including how staff will be accounted for.

Designating a central meeting place is useful for checking in on staff and having them account for the patients, that they are all out of the building before staff are sent home. Procedures for evacuating patients with disabilities and limited mobility without elevators should be considered. EOPs should also address the facility's infrastructure, with procedures for shutting down critical operations, such as disabling any central oxygen or medical gas system.

Anticipated Storm Disaster: Hurricane Katrina In New Orleans

The story of Hurricane Katrina in New Orleans shows how important planning is for meeting patient needs, and how sometimes disasters are beyond the scope of what planners anticipated. This disaster affected multiple states and devastated the healthcare system in New Orleans, unlike anything that had ever been experienced by other US healthcare systems.

All but three hospitals in the city experienced severe damage, and some were completely destroyed. Physical access to the remaining facilities was almost impossible because of the flooding. The response to the storm and the subsequent flooding was not adequate and provided many lessons to healthcare professionals and planners. Subsequent federal legislation required significant improvements to planning for future healthcare responses at the federal, state, and local levels. That is why this is such an important case to study.

Disaster Strikes

In the summer of 2005, 16 city hospitals were providing inpatient and outpatient care to the people of New Orleans and the surrounding area. New Orleans was the center for the state's public health system. Charity Hospital was the primary source of healthcare for a largely poor and uninsured population that suffered from high rates of chronic diseases, such as heart disease and diabetes. Charity Hospital had one of the busiest emergency departments in the state.

Hurricane Katrina struck the Gulf Coast of Florida on Thursday, August 25, and the next day, in anticipation of its arrival, the governor of Louisiana declared a state of emergency, urging communities and cities to prepare. The city of New Orleans, located about six feet below sea level, is surrounded by water and is protected by levees. On Saturday, the mayor called for voluntary evacuation, allowing residents in low-lying areas to get out first. He designated the Louisiana Superdome, which was located at one of the city's higher elevations, as a shelter for evacuees with nowhere else to go. As the governor and mayor learned of the coming storm's intensity, the governor sent a letter requesting a presidential disaster declaration, which was issued. On Sunday, the mayor declared mandatory evacuations—a first for New Orleans.

Early on Monday, August 29, 2005, the hurricane hit New Orleans, and, one by one, levees around the city began to overflow or break. Flooding

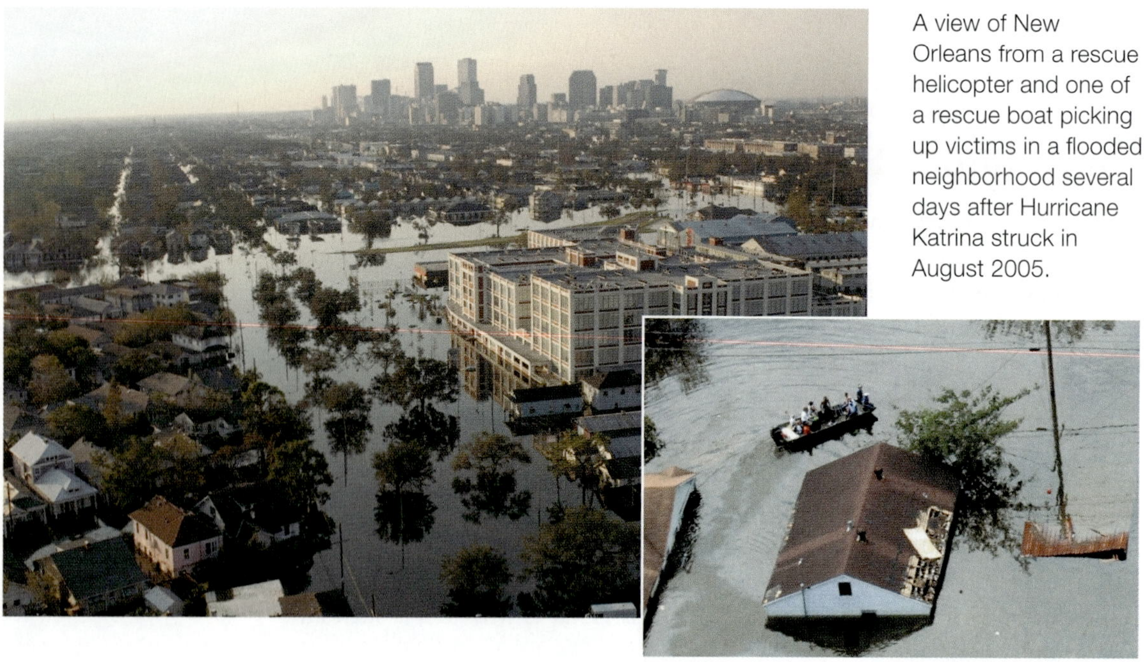

A view of New Orleans from a rescue helicopter and one of a rescue boat picking up victims in a flooded neighborhood several days after Hurricane Katrina struck in August 2005.

occurred in 80% of the city. That day, the president issued a declaration calling Louisiana, Mississippi, and Alabama major disaster areas.

Approximately 1,800 people lost their lives during Katrina and its aftermath. After the hurricane, an estimated three million people were without electricity. More than one million people evacuated and spread across the US, housed by family, friends, and shelters.

Communication and Coordination Difficulties

Communication was one of the greatest obstacles facing the city and the medical community. Working equipment and standard communication protocols were lacking. The infrastructure for landline phones was destroyed. The majority of cell phones were inoperable because they could not be recharged, or the cellular signals were jammed and calls were dropped. Satellite communications were unreliable.

The mayor and governor struggled with communications in coordinating resources from the Federal Emergency Management Agency (FEMA), National Guard, US military, nonprofit disaster response organizations, businesses, and religious congregations. Many times, the efforts of one group were stalled by waiting for permission or direction, or they got in the way of efficiently carrying out the duties of another group.

Evacuation

When the hurricane was approaching, hospitals discharged many patients, but the sickest remained. Hospital and nursing home administrators in potential danger zones had to decide whether or not to evacuate their patients since evacuations are risky, difficult, and expensive.

The large-scale city evacuations began on September 1. Many rescue boats had washed away and the availability of personnel, such as the National Guard, to help move people was limited, so evacuation was slow. Victims from shelters and from failing healthcare facilities were evacuated to a temporary field hospital at the Louis Armstrong New Orleans International Airport. The medical response teams at the airport were overwhelmed, as they evaluated 4,000 evacuees to determine who needed medical attention. The teams prioritized and prepared victims requiring treatment or ongoing care for airlift to healthcare facilities outside the flood zone.

Without a reliable method of communication, the functioning hospitals did not know whether more patients would be arriving or whether they should send medical teams to other areas. Once the levees broke and the floodwaters rushed in, the hospitals and medical centers of New Orleans needed to evacuate if they could. The challenges were far greater than during

Expand Your Knowledge

Local radio communications had also been knocked out, so air traffic control was limited or nonexistent in some air spaces. Rescue helicopter and plane pilots, from the National Guard, US military, and volunteers, had to work together in hazardous, low-flying conditions without the usual air traffic assistance. They played a key role in the rescue and hospital evacuation efforts.

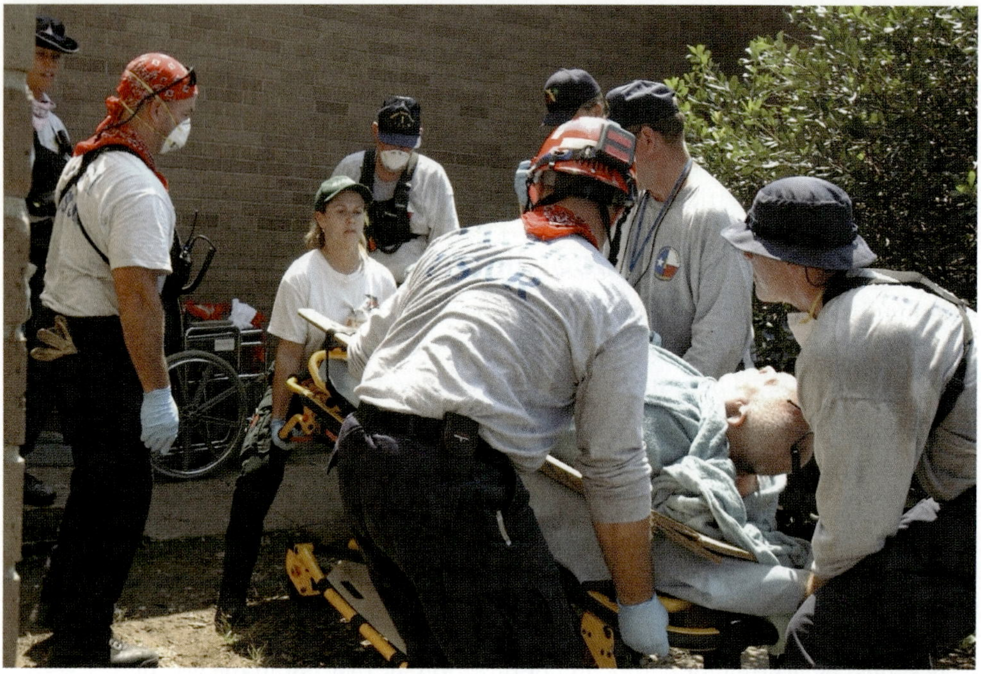

On August 31, 2005, members of a FEMA Urban Search and Rescue (USAR) team evacuate patients from a New Orleans nursing home facility.

Hurricane Ivan the year before. Because there were no functioning elevators in the flooded hospitals, patients had to be carried down stairs, together with their monitoring equipment and intravenous bags.

Facilities that had evacuated patients in preparation for Hurricane Ivan used buses and semitrailer trucks equipped with air-conditioning and generators. During the Katrina response, they were unable to access these vehicles because so many roads were flooded. Fuel and rental cars were in short supply, and many forms of public transportation had been shut down. When available, patients were put into heavy-duty National Guard vehicles that could go through shallow waters or boats and then transferred to ambulances that took them to the airport. Some patients were taken by helicopter to Florida and Texas. Before Katrina's landfall, 19 nursing homes evacuated their residents. Once the flooding began, an additional 32 homes did the same. Administrators at St. Rita's Nursing Home decided to wait out the storm. As a result, 35 people died there.

The administrators of many healthcare facilities thought that they were prepared to handle the hurricane because they did not anticipate the flooding from broken levees. Those facilities that remained open had great difficulty maintaining expected standards of care. In hospitals that lost power, pulmonary ventilator systems and other medical equipment requiring electricity did not work. Most hospitals lacked an adequate supply of water safe to drink, safe food, and medications. These shortages lasted for days.

Compounding the problems were staff shortages. Many healthcare workers were evacuated or forced to leave the area because their homes had been destroyed. Incapacitated in terms of equipment and without supplies, hospitals struggled to provide care and keep patients alive until help arrived. Many medical staff members worked 18-hour days. Because of the heroic efforts of the healthcare personnel, most patients survived, but an estimated 215 people died in New Orleans hospitals and nursing homes as a result of the failure to evacuate.

Heroes Corner

Hospital Staff Struggle to Keep Patients Alive in Charity Hospital

Before Hurricane Katrina struck, New Orleans's Charity Hospital was the largest public hospital in the US. Though the hospital suffered some initial damage, the emergency generators in the basement provided power when most of the city had none. However, by Tuesday morning, August 30, the hospital's basement was flooded, shutting down the generators. Soon the water reached the 1st floor. The flooding trapped about 360 patients and 1,200 staff members. The temperature soared to 110° F with high humidity.

Without running water and power, hospital staff could not wash their hands or use the laboratory, monitors, X-ray machines, and operating room. Fortunately, the hospital had 10 portable diesel-powered generators and a few hands-free ventilators to try to maintain patient care on some level.

The staff moved 40 to 50 patients from the first floor ED to the second-floor auditorium. They had to strap patients who were manually ventilated to backboards and carry them up the stairs. They also lugged the supplies. Throughout the rest of the hospital, the staff assessed patient conditions. The water around the facility was chest deep. They used a boat to transport the sickest patients, to the Tulane Medical Center's helipad, and then had to get the patients to the top of its parking garage. Once there, the patients and staff with them had to watch and wait as patients and staff from Tulane Medical Center were evacuated first.

By the fifth day after the storm, only 100 patients had been evacuated from Charity Hospital. The staff had been rationing their food and using intravenous fluids to keep themselves hydrated in the intense heat. They had found diesel fuel for the generators in an abandoned ambulance. When airboats and trucks finally came, it took only three and a half hours to evacuate the hospital. The hospital staff had managed to keep all but eight people alive during the five-day ordeal.

For an account of a doctor's memories and the solutions the staff found for some challenges, read the article at **http://EmDPrp2.ParadigmEducation.com/NEJM**.

Web

The Federal Healthcare Response

After the President issued a disaster declaration for Louisiana on Monday, August 29, the US Department of Health and Human Services activated the National Disaster Medical System (NDMS) and sent in emergency medical teams, shelters, portable medical units, pharmaceuticals, and supplies. The Disaster Medical Assistant Teams (DMATs) transferred patients from hospitals in flooded areas to hospitals located out of the area.

The NDMS also sent medical teams to provide care and assistance to the few hospitals that were still functioning. These self-sufficient teams came in mobile medical units that provided enough medical equipment and supplies, large tents, generators, and other support equipment necessary to be self-sufficient for up to three days and treat up to 250 patients per day. The OR-2 DMAT (Oregon-2 DMAT) was deployed for 11 days. The OR-2 DMAT team members also became fatigued because they operated with limited medical supplies, inadequate food and water, intermittent electricity, and no air-conditioning. Medical personnel who were stationed at the airport worked as many as 60 hours without sleep.

The Medical Reserve Corps, run by the Office of the Surgeon General at the time, linked its database of healthcare professionals with state databases

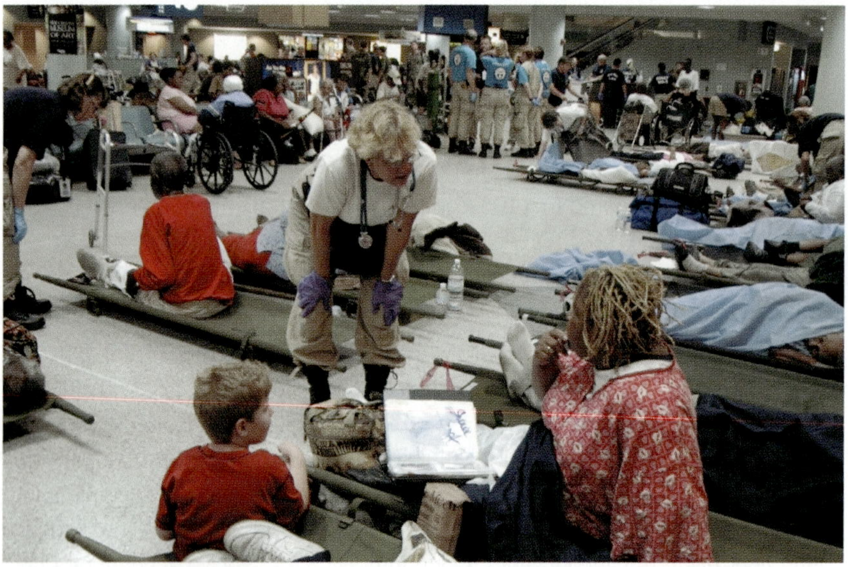

Evacuees and patients arrive at the Louis Armstrong New Orleans International Airport where FEMA Disaster Medical Assistance Teams (DMATs) set up operations immediately after Hurricane Katrina struck in August 31, 2005. The DMATs come from around the US. The evacuees are given food, water, and medical attention.

to confirm the **credentials**, or proof of education and professional skills, of the volunteers. The MRC volunteers were urged to work with preexisting rescue teams and not act independently.

The Centers for Disease Control and Prevention (CDC) provided millions of doses of vaccines for influenza, tetanus and diphtheria, hepatitis A, and hepatitis B. People handling the storage and distribution of the vaccines had difficulty keeping them refrigerated at the correct temperature, which is essential for vaccine safety and effectiveness.

Patient Overflow to Other Areas

Patients who could not get care in New Orleans sought medical services at other area hospitals. Our Lady of the Lake Regional Medical Center, in Baton Rouge, Louisiana, operated at full capacity and hospitalized over 80 displaced patients. All staff members at the hospital worked overtime, often not going home. Some staff filled in for coworkers who could not get to work. The hospital set up a 24-hour child-care center. Medical and other supplies did not arrive until several days after the storm.

Before Katrina, the ED of nearby West Jefferson Medical Center, 15 minutes from downtown New Orleans in Marrero, Louisiana, saw an average of 180 patients a day. Immediately after the storm, the hospital saw as many as 600 patients a day, mostly for nonemergency conditions. The most common problems were wound infections, gastrointestinal problems, dysentery, and dehydration due to lack of safe drinking water. Bacteria, toxins, and chemicals had mixed with floodwaters, causing health problems. The number of ED patients requiring hospitalization jumped by 40 percent overnight.

Loss of Medical Records

Most hospitals were still using paper medical records when Hurricane Katrina occurred. The storm and flooding destroyed millions of pages of medical records in hospitals, clinics, medical offices, and pharmacies. Thousands of patients had to depend on their memory and knowledge of their medical and medication history when they sought care, leading to difficulties and delays in treatment.

A few New Orleans hospitals, including the US Department of Veterans Affairs (VA) facilities and Kindred Hospital, had electronic medical records. The VA had backed up its medical records off-site and was able to electronically send the full medical records to facilities caring for transferred patients.

The loss of medical records sparked some innovative solutions. With help from public and private groups, the federal government established a website where healthcare workers treating evacuees could retrieve some prescription histories and other health information. The website was assembled by bringing together existing databases from retail pharmacies and government health programs, such as Medicaid.

When the Harris Health System created a large clinic at the Houston Astrodome in Texas for evacuees, it included 80 computer terminals for registering patients and recording their medical histories and information. Volunteers in Houston registered and documented patient information for 8,000 evacuees, creating new electronic medical records.

Some health information professionals also found innovative solutions, by backing up records on laptop computers, flash drives, or handheld devices. One nurse practitioner from New Orleans stored the medical records for 100 homebound, elderly patients on her PalmPilot. After her patients evacuated, she received calls from providers from across the US who were treating them. She was able to download and fax the medical history and lab work for these patients to wherever the information was needed.

Equipment and Supply Shortages

Immediately following the hurricane, there was a heavy demand for medical supplies in the region, although few demands could be met. Cardinal Health, one of the main distributors of hospital supplies, was damaged and closed its distribution center. As a result, supplies that were usually provided locally had to be brought in from Alabama, Georgia, and Texas. Because of security concerns, medical products had to be escorted by local and state authorities.

Once hospitals were able to procure supplies, they ordered two to three times the usual amount because they expected to care for many more patients. Typical requests included water; generators; emergency items such as flashlights, linens and cots; and medical supplies, including antibiotics, antibiotic soap, gowns, drapes, and surgical instruments.

Additional Healthcare System Challenges

Soon after the hurricane, a temporary ED and medical clinic opened at New Orleans's Ernest N. Morial Convention Center. Four mobile clinics were set up. Attempts were also made to open clinics in well-known community places, such as schools. However, healthcare professionals often had difficulty getting to these clinics because physical access was blocked in some areas, and civil disorder was a problem in others.

In addition, New Orleans was unprepared to evacuate and provide medical care for patients who had difficulty taking care of themselves or understanding the implications of what might be happening. These patients had what are termed **access and functional needs**. These people did not require hospitalization, but their conditions required care that, at the time, could not be appropriately provided in a general shelter as they had difficulties caring for themselves. To complicate the problem, the various agencies and departments that had responsibility for the care of these 45,000 patients could not agree on which patients had these access and functional needs.

When employers did not reopen their businesses after the hurricane, many people lost their health insurance. People also had difficulty locating their usual doctors or connecting with new ones. They could not find open pharmacies or pay for medical care and medications. Many people with chronic illnesses experienced complications because they had no access to essential medications and treatments, such as oxygen, insulin, or kidney dialysis.

Recovery and Rebuilding

The devastation of Hurricane Katrina helped New Orleans rebuild its healthcare system with a new approach—where hospitals are supported with public health centers in the neighborhoods. The city has built more than 60 clinics dispersed throughout the city's residential neighborhoods. The local clinics focus on prevention and delivering primary care services for the uninsured. All of the clinics use electronic medical records. Some clinics work with special populations, such as teenagers, musicians, or the homeless.

Louisiana also received grant money to develop a health information exchange. All information for patients seen in New Orleans and Baton Rouge was entered into this system. Any provider in this area could look up their patients' medical history and list of medications.

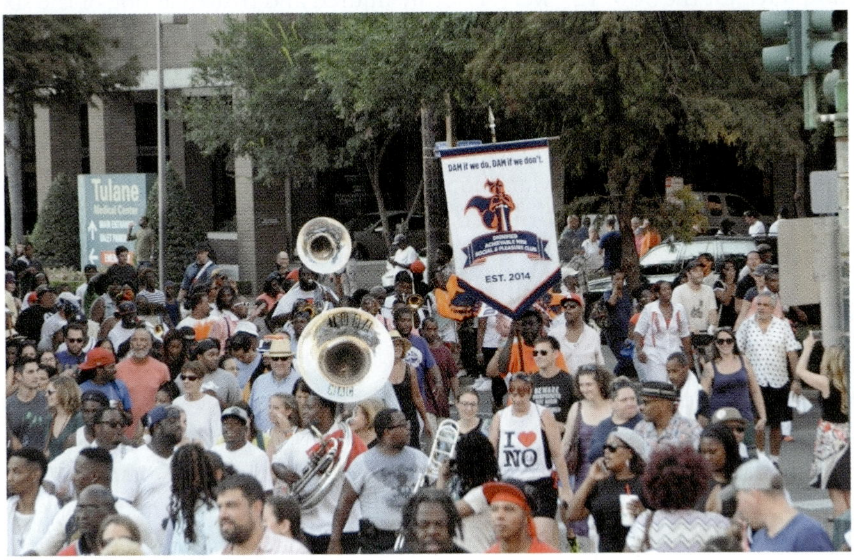

On the ten-year anniversary of Hurricane Katrina on August 29, 2015, a New Orleans brass band parade marches past the repaired Tulane Medical Center.

As for Charity Hospital, it is currently being renovated for new uses. For those residents needing hospital care, a new state-of-the-art facility, the University Medical Center, delivers the latest medical services to the city's entire community.

Mass Casualties: The 2013 Boston Marathon Bombings

In an emergency, the first challenge is knowing what has occurred and what kind and level of response are needed. Sometimes, a healthcare facility receives notification and other times a healthcare facility's first sign that something tragic has happened is when victims show up for treatment. The local authorities may not be able to provide complete information to the healthcare facility (about what to expect in terms of the number and types of victims or duration of the incident), because the event may still be unfolding.

The explosions at the Boston Marathon required a rapid response from the entire healthcare system in the Boston area, because there was a surge of patients who experienced severe trauma. On April 15, 2013 at 2:49 p.m., two homemade bombs exploded within 12 seconds of each other, 210 yards from the finish line of the Boston Marathon on Boylston Street. The homemade bombs consisted of pressure cookers filled with nails, ball bearings, and screws. The devices exploded in the middle of a crowd of thousands of runners, families, friends, and spectators.

Be Aware

Level I trauma centers have the specially trained medical staff and equipment needed to care for people who are seriously injured.

Three people were killed. Almost 300 were injured and treated at 27 local hospitals. Of the 300, 127 were seriously injured and treated at one of the six Level I trauma centers in Boston.

Preparing for the Race

The response capabilities were determined in great part by the preparation for the race. The Boston Marathon attracts 30,000 runners annually, and generally more than 1,000 runners, fans, and bystanders receive care each year for medical issues that go along with such a long and grueling race. These issues include overheating, exhaustion, dehydration, and cardiac and respiratory problems.

Every year, many agencies and groups, including federal, state, and local public safety, public health and EMS personnel, and the Boston Athletic Association, work together to prepare for the event. Their emergency and disaster preparedness includes a tabletop exercise where they practice their response to potential scenarios that might occur during the marathon. As part of the city's long-standing planning, Boston's EMS personnel were

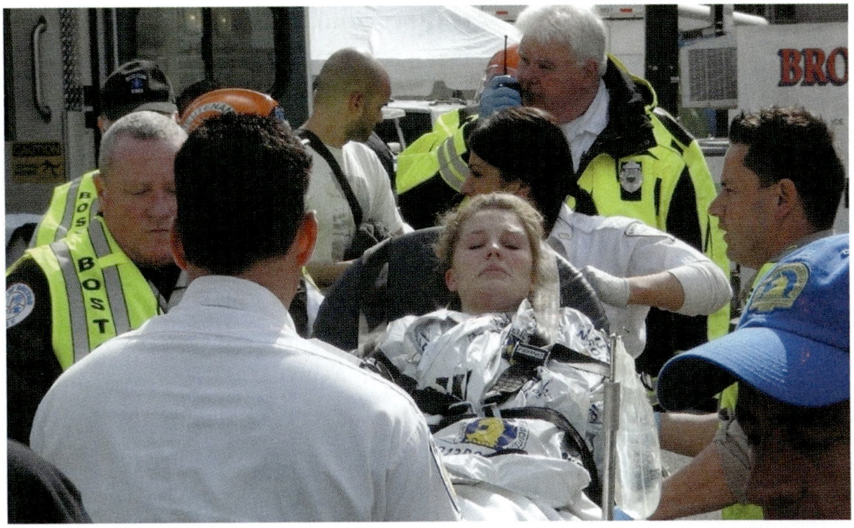

On April 15, first responders and Boston Marathon medical teams move swiftly to take care of the victims and get them to treatment.

trained to use tourniquets (which are constricting or compressing devices) to control severe bleeding. The medical system for the race included 26 medical tents placed along the course and 2 near the finish line. The tent closest to the finish line was named Alpha Medical Tent.

Initial Medical Response

Within seconds after the bombs exploded, first responders (police, fire, and EMS), medical volunteers from the Alpha Medical Tent, those watching the marathon, and other volunteers began to care for the injured. One key action was to apply tourniquets to stop the severe bleeding. The Alpha Medical Tent formed teams and initiated a mass casualty response. They used the tent as a **casualty collection point**, the place to bring patients to sort them by category of injury, stabilize their medical conditions, and then send them to hospitals for care.

All injured patients were transported from Boylston Street within 45 minutes from the time of the bomb blast. Every patient who was transported to a hospital survived because of the lifesaving care they received at the scene, in the ambulances, and at the hospital.

> **Expand Your Knowledge**
>
> The American College of Emergency Physicians provides resources, such as webinars and toolkits for emergency department and hospital personnel. The following relate to bombings and resulting injuries: http://EmDPrp2.ParadigmEducation.com/ACEPSurge and http://EmDPrp2.ParadigmEducation.com/ACEPInjury.
>
> Web

Hospitals Activate Emergency Operation Plans

The trauma centers at the city's hospitals received notification of the explosions via phone calls and from personal twitter feeds. The hospitals immediately activated their emergency operations plans. Each issued its designated code to let the hospital staff know about the emergency. The on-call radiology staff for emergencies were notified. Patients who were in the emergency

Expand Your Knowledge

For more information, watch these two YouTube interviews with staff responders at Massachusetts General Hospital sharing their experiences on April 15, 2013: http://EmDPrp2.ParadigmEducation.com/MassGenFirstResponders http://EmDPrp2.ParadigmEducation.com/MassGenCommunity.

departments (EDs) at the time were either admitted and transferred to inpatient units or discharged home to make room for the incoming wounded.

The doctors encountered physical injuries common to bombs exploding close to the ground: legs amputated by the blast; open fractures in the leg, thigh, and pelvis; burns; injuries to the head and organs in the abdomen; and projectiles imbedded in tissue.

In the city's trauma hospitals, many of the operating rooms were fully scheduled at the time of the blasts. Elective surgeries were put on hold or canceled. One hospital, Massachusetts General, treated 31 blast victims in an hour. Five critically injured patients were transferred into the operating room within approximately eight minutes of one another. This was possible because the hospitals had comprehensive plans for emergencies and disasters. They had also tested these plans through exercises.

Heroes Corner

Racing to Meet the Needs

During the 2013 Boston Marathon, Massachusetts General Hospital had a team running in the marathon. This team was founded by Dr. Howard Weinstein to support the Pediatric Hematology-Oncology Department. He was at mile 25 when he heard the first bomb go off near the finish line.

Dr. Weinstein and other members of the marathon team returned to the hospital immediately to care for the wounded. Dr. David King, a surgeon on the team, went directly from the race to the operating room, working straight for 30 hours until all the necessary surgeries had been completed.

Every member of the hospital staff exhibited similar dedication.

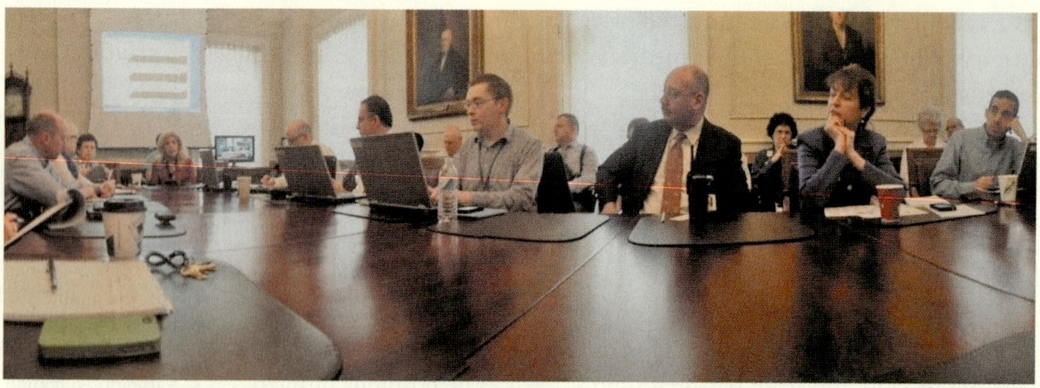

With notice of the bombings, the senior vice president of surgical and anesthesia services set off the emergency signal and established a hospital emergency operations center in the Trustees Room.

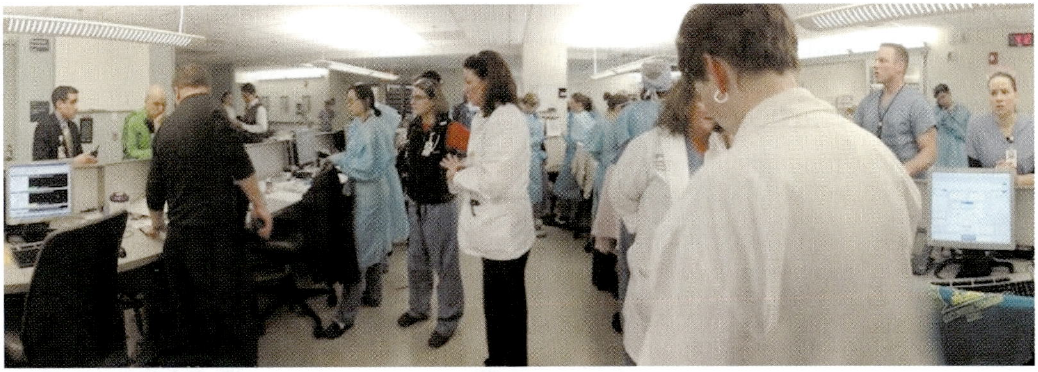

The alert went out during shift-change at Massachusetts General Hospital, doubling the available staff. The ED rapidly cleared its occupied patient bays, transported routine admissions to other care units, and received assistance from colleagues arriving to help manage the medical surge. ED Incident Commander Dr. Paul Biddinger can be seen at his post (in black on left).

Information Obstacles to Overcome

Information systems in EDs are critical to ensure everyone providing care knows what is happening to patients in real time. However, in the case of the Boston Marathon bombing, when patients first arrived in the hospital EDs, hospital staff did not know who they were. The staff had to find a way to identify each person to record the doctors' assessment of that patient's condition, and which tests and procedures had been ordered. The first challenge was how to give a name to a patient whose identity was not known. This is called the **unidentified patient naming convention** (naming convention).

At Brigham and Women's Hospital, the registration supervisor anticipated this problem. As the EMTs and paramedics brought patients in, the registration staff placed unidentified trauma packets on each stretcher. For each patient, they created a unique letter combination (XYZ) for the first name and wrote UNIDENTIFIED for the last name. Furthermore, they had a tracking board that indicated the location of each patient, and tiles listing the unique letter combination for each unidentified patient were placed on the tracking board. However, it still became difficult to distinguish the patients on the tracking board with the limited information on the tiles.

The physician orders for tests and procedures were entered into each patient's electronic medical record. However, because of problems with the naming convention, there was confusion. Some tests were ordered more than once for the same patient by different doctors. Radiologists had difficulty determining which tests had been completed and which were duplicate orders. Some orders were canceled because they did not know which patients

Be Aware

Three victims died at the scene of the blast, but every patient (almost 300) delivered to a hospital survived. The high survival rate was due to the presence of medical teams at the marathon, exceptional first responder reactions, hospitals that effectively applied their emergency operation plans, and dedicated, knowledgeable staff who improvised solutions for resource limitations as needed.

Be Aware

Injuries from explosions, known as **blast injuries**, occur from the pressure of the blast itself, the flying debris, being thrown back from the blast, or any fire that develops.

had received orders for tests. This confusion made it difficult for secretaries and radiology technologists to do their jobs.

Radiology Rises to the Challenges

The radiology departments made a significant contribution to sorting through the confusion and handling the medical surge. The radiology teams faced many challenges. They had to gather enough available equipment and doctors and technologists to perform the large volume of X-rays, **computed tomography (CT)** scans, and ultrasounds. They had to enter many new medical orders into the computer at once, and communicate the results swiftly and accurately to staff. The staff quickly modified the usual procedures to address the issues while the emergency was happening.

Be Aware

CT scanners use X-rays to take detailed images inside the human body. The images appear as sequential image slices of each organ being X-rayed. All of the images are saved as a group on a computer.

Brigham and Women's Hospital, a Level I trauma center, typically had only two to three emergency radiologists available. Once the radiology department heard about the bombings, an additional nine radiology physicians and technologists from the inpatient and outpatient units were called in to help.

On normal days, the ED had one CT scanner, two portable X-ray machines that could be moved from bed to bed, two computerized X-ray machines in another location, and an ultrasound machine. The radiologists located three additional CT scanners in other hospital units and brought in a third portable X-ray machine.

The usual process for taking X-rays was quickly found to be too time-consuming with the number of critically injured patients and limited number of portable X-ray machines. Instead, the emergency physicians and trauma surgeons used the three ultrasound machines to do what is known as **focused assessments with sonography for trauma (FAST)** for internal examinations. The use of the portable ultrasound machines also proved critical in diagnosis.

A Closer Look

Adapting the Work Process

The Brigham and Women's Hospital ED received 29 patients in the first 30 minutes after the bombing. To diagnose and treat each patient quickly, the physicians decided to use ultrasound at each patient's stretcher. Because there was not enough time for a complete documentation of the results, one doctor wrote down the results of the ultrasound on a piece of paper, which was then taped to each patient's stretcher.

Within the ED, to avoid difficulties in matching patients with their CT scan results, two radiology trainees were placed near the CT scanner so that they could immediately communicate the results to the emergency medicine physicians and trauma surgery team. They also used the telephone to call members of the team located in other parts of the hospital.

The Emergency Code Ends

After approximately four hours, the Boston hospitals realized that they would not be receiving any other injured patients from the bombings. The hospital incident command center deactivated their emergency codes, yet the disaster response was still not done. While emergency surgeries continued, the personnel not involved in those surgeries, and who came from other areas of the hospital, were sent to the inpatient areas where they were most needed. Extraordinary care continued for the patients, family members, friends, and staff long after April 15, 2013.

In addition to providing medical care, Massachusetts General used the Blum Patient and Family Learning Center as a family assistance center, providing support and information for the victims' loved ones. The facility and its chaplaincy department later set up support groups for the staff. Similar accommodations were set up at other responding hospitals.

Expand Your Knowledge

For an analysis of the emergency response by Boston and Massachusetts state authorities, read "After Action Report for the Response to the 2013 Boston Marathon Bombings" at http://EmDPrp2.ParadigmEducation.com/AfterActionReport.

An Emerging Infection: Ebola in Texas

Specialized credentials are required for laboratories to conduct testing on human specimens that might be hazardous. This can make preparing for and diagnosing patients with signs of an emerging infectious disease challenging, as the following example demonstrates.

In December 2013, an outbreak of the **Ebola Virus Disease (EVD)** started in Liberia and spread to other West African countries. EVD is a rare and highly infectious disease transmitted through bodily fluids. As many as 50%–60% of those who contract the virus die. EVD is spread when one person comes in direct contact with the body fluids of an infected person or through contaminated needles. Infected body fluids include blood, urine, sweat, semen, and breast milk.

EVD is diagnosed through specialized laboratory testing of blood specimens. Before 2014, only a few US laboratories located at federal agencies were given permission to conduct this testing, which had not yet been approved by the **US Food and Drug Administration (FDA)**. EVD is considered a **select agent**—a biological or chemical substance that has been identified as having the potential to pose a severe threat to public health and safety. Select agents require special **assays**, or laboratory testing procedures.

Be Aware

The Association of Public Health Laboratories reports that 42 million diagnostic and medical tests are performed daily across the US.

The **Department of Defense (DoD)** had developed an assay for a specialized EVD test, but only a limited number of testing kits were available and very few laboratories in the nation were allowed to use them. Labs had to show proficiency in running the test before they were approved to receive the restricted number of testing kits and test specimens.

Be Aware

There are also veterinary labs run by the USDA that conduct animal testing to try to determine the first sign of diseases shared by humans and animals.

Laboratory Response Network

Since 1999, the CDC has partnered with the Federal Bureau of Investigation and the Association of Public Health Laboratories to form the **Laboratory Response Network (LRN)**. This network of state and local public health, federal, and military laboratories responds to any infectious disease, bioterrorist, or chemical threats. The LRN organizes the laboratories into a three-level system. Each level of laboratories conducts more sophisticated testing than the previous level.

The first-level laboratories, known as **sentinel laboratories**, are the hospital, clinic, or private labs where most laboratory technicians work and where most medical testing is conducted. A sentinel laboratory may be the first laboratory to detect a possible biological or chemical agent. A positive result in a test is considered a **presumptive result**, meaning that confirmatory tests are still needed. The lab then alerts public health authorities and refers suspicious specimens to the next level of laboratory, which is the reference laboratory. (National and international regulations require that infectious materials be properly packaged and labeled before they are shipped.)

Reference laboratories have the reagents and technology necessary to conduct more sophisticated tests for identifying or confirming biological and chemical agents. Reference labs include state and local public health, veterinary, and military laboratories as well as food, water, and environmental testing labs. All reference laboratories in the LRN use the same protocols, reagents, and equipment and process specimens in the same way. Thus, the result of any test is the same in Texas and in any LRN lab in the US, including the labs at the CDC.

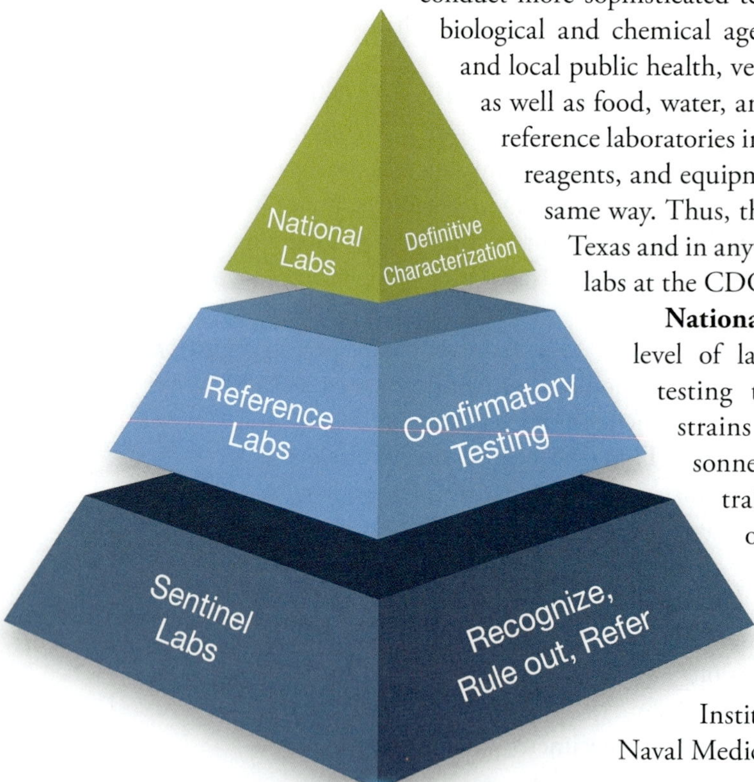

National laboratories are the highest level of laboratories, capable of advanced testing to isolate and identify specific strains of disease agents, having personnel with special credentials and training to test for highly dangerous and infectious Category A biological agents, such as EVD. National laboratories include labs operated by the CDC, US Army Medical Research Institute for Infectious Diseases, and Naval Medical Research Center.

Preparing the Laboratories for Testing for EVD

In the spring and early summer of 2014, the laboratories in state departments of health (DOHs) began hearing about EVD in West Africa. First the information appeared in emailed information circulated through public health LISTSERVs. Then the CDC started educating hospital and other healthcare professionals about the symptoms, and members of the LRN were informed of a specialized test for EVD and the protocols to test for the presence of this infectious disease.

Be Aware

A LISTSERV is an electronic mailing list to which people subscribe. People join LISTSERVs to receive information about a topic of interest.

When physicians initially suspect that a patient has an emerging infectious disease, a sample of the blood needs to go through a specialized blood test for diagnosis. For emerging diseases, the test may not yet have been approved by the FDA for general use by healthcare systems. The FDA, though, can issue an **Emergency Use Authorization** to allow the special use of medical products, such as specialized blood tests, to diagnose or treat serious life-threatening diseases when there are no available alternatives.

By early August 2014, the threat seemed pressing enough that the FDA issued an Emergency Use Authorization to the DoD to allow about a dozen LRN labs located near international airports to conduct the tests and receive the testing kits.

Dallas/Fort Worth International Airport is a major hub for international flights. The Texas **Department of State Health Services (DSHS)** was notified to prepare for potential cases of EVD, and the lab director of the DSHS reference laboratory was approached about testing for EVD. The lab director discussed this with the commissioner of the DSHS because it was controversial to prepare to conduct testing for EVD before there were US cases of the disease. When the commissioner agreed, the DSHS's Austin lab received one of the kits.

Although the lab had not tested for this organism before, laboratory technicians were familiar with the testing method and technology. The procedures for processing the specimen, though, were slightly different, and the chemical **reagent** (or specialized reacting assay substance) was specific for detecting EVD.

Before the lab could receive specimens and start testing, the lab director had a lot of work to do to educate the technicians and other staff in the lab and throughout the state. Because of concerns about EVD, the director wanted the laboratory staff to understand that the technicians conducting the tests would be highly trained and competent to handle this highly infectious material to prevent causing any fear. She began a series of communications with staff and officials at state, county, and local agencies.

Epidemiologists (public health professionals who track the spread of disease) from the DSHS met with the management staff of the laboratory and its **Biothreat Team**, the team designated for testing specimens that might pose a biological threat. They agreed on the safety procedures and how everyone would communicate requests for testing and reporting the results. Any positive result from a test would need to be communicated quickly and to many partners.

By mid-August 2014, the DSHS lab had received the Ebola testing kit from the DoD and passed the **external quality assurance review**, which is an evaluation of a laboratory conducted by an official assessor outside the lab, which is the required specialized credential. All members of the Biothreat Team were extensively trained on the procedures until everyone felt comfortable performing the test. The process for the new test was similar to testing that the Biothreat Team members had previously performed, so they were able to quickly implement the test.

To prevent exposure to the Ebola virus, the team members would wear **personal protective equipment (PPE)**, or gowns, goggles, gloves, masks, and special respiratory protection. The laboratory also had to make sure that it had the necessary **biosafety protocols**, or safety procedures for handling highly infectious biological materials, appropriate for testing EVD. One safety step was to remove all glass in the testing lab to prevent any glass being broken and potentially tearing the PPE. By August 26, 2014, the laboratory staff was ready to begin receiving specimens for EVD testing.

First Case of Ebola Virus Disease in the US

In late September 2014, the **index patient**, or first medically identified patient in the US, traveled from Liberia to Dallas. Mr. Duncan did not feel ill when he left Liberia and did not develop fully identifiable symptoms until approximately four days after arriving in Texas. He sought help at Texas Health Presbyterian Hospital, Dallas. Because of his symptoms and his recent international travel, the hospital reached out to the CDC for advice on how to diagnose and treat him. The CDC recommended testing for EVD. The

A Closer Look

Shipping Biological Specimens

Biological specimens can be shipped if properly packaged and labeled. They require special documentation and packaging materials that meet regulations of the Department of Transportation and the International Air Transport Association. Highly infectious specimens require **triple packaging**. Specimens are placed in a plastic bag with absorbent material within a hard-plastic container that is leak proof. That container is placed in another container with dry ice or cold packs to keep the specimen frozen or at 4° C.

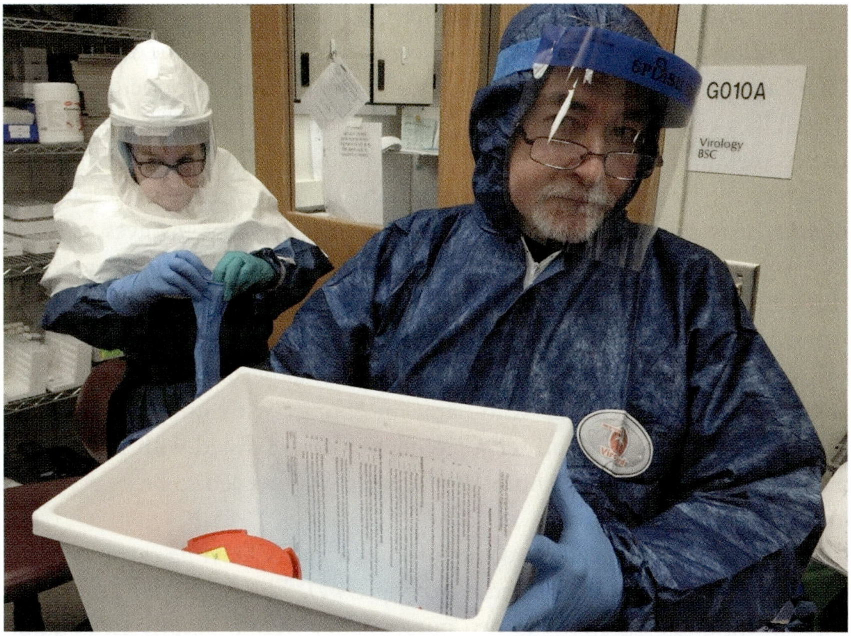

This CDC photo demonstrates the proper procedure for transporting biological samples from a patient suspected to have EVD (foreground) and donning personal protective equipment (background).

hospital isolated the patient and contacted the head epidemiologist at the Dallas County Department of Health (DOH). Personnel from the county DOH, Texas DSHS, CDC, and the hospital coordinated with one another throughout the process.

Two sets of blood specimens were drawn from the patient, one for the reference laboratory at Austin, Texas, and one for the national laboratory at the CDC. The Dallas County LRN sent lab personnel to Texas Health Presbyterian Hospital, Dallas, to ensure that the first sample was properly packaged. On September 29, they sent the specimens through FedEx to both the DSHS lab in Austin and to the CDC.

Testing Begins

The morning of Tuesday, September 30, 2014, the DSHS staff was lined up to get their annual flu shots when the call came that the package was on its way. When it arrived at 9:07 a.m., the Biothreat Team was waiting. A similar package also arrived at the CDC at about the same time. It took three hours to run the tests, and both the Austin and the CDC labs completed testing at about the same time. At the Austin lab, there was shock at the results. It was EVD!

The day before, the CDC and the DSHS, working with their public information offices, had agreed on how to communicate the results. The CDC and the DSHS informed the commissioner of health immediately, and the CDC and the DSHS made the public announcement of the positive test results together.

Once the first case of EVD was diagnosed, county, state, and CDC epidemiologists conducted **contact tracing**. Contact tracing involves tracking down and monitoring every person who may have been exposed to EVD through contact with the index patient. A similar process would be done when other patients develop the disease. The county health department took the lead and performed contact tracing for hospital personnel, Mr. Duncan's acquaintances, and anyone who came in contact with him while he was symptomatic. The state and CDC epidemiologists assisted with the investigation because of the large number of people who needed to be interviewed and monitored.

Two nurses had already become infected with EVD while caring for Mr. Duncan before he was suspected of having EVD. The Austin lab conducted the confirmatory tests for the two nurses. They were promptly treated and later recovered. Hundreds of people who had potential contact with the three EVD patients were monitored for signs of the disease for 21 days. None of the people who were monitored developed EVD.

For several weeks after the initial testing, the DSHS Biothreat Team received blood specimens for people who had been potentially exposed, at all hours. The staff developed a plan to conduct the needed testing and allow time for those doing the testing to rest between tests. The Texas Medical Operations Center provided support for testing supplies and specimen delivery.

When the Austin lab did not have enough PPE for the Biothreat Team because the items were on back order from the vendor, the San Antonio and Houston LRN labs sent cases of biosafety hoods. In mid-October, the Dallas County LRN lab joined the Austin lab in conducting testing for EVD. Like the Austin lab, the Dallas lab would receive many requests for EVD testing. This EVD case study was one where all those involved—the hospital, laboratories, departments of health, and the CDC—worked effectively together in a coordinated response to this emerging infection.

All three of the case studies provided in this chapter--a health system response to a natural disaster, a multi-casualty incident resulting from a terrorist event, and a laboratory and health system response to an emerging infectious disease--prove key lessons in both what was done well and what problems arose. Each are useful in illustrating how health professionals can prepare for disasters and strategies for responding effectively.

Chapter Summary

Healthcare facilities have special requirements from the government and The Joint Commission that also mandate that they conduct comprehensive emergency management planning and use an ICS structure adapted to healthcare. One of the requirements is that hospitals must have regular drills to test for their readiness for emergencies and disasters. They also must have a backup source of power and an evacuation plan.

During and after disasters, healthcare facilities may be overwhelmed with victims seeking medical care. Facilities may be damaged or unable to operate. Facilities will often experience shortages of supplies if the aftermath of a disaster disrupts normal shipping and deliveries. Additionally, facilities may experience staff shortages and loss of medical records.

In 2005, Hurricane Katrina and the floods that followed the storm taxed the healthcare system of New Orleans in ways that had rarely been experienced in the US. Many people were saved through rescue, evacuation, and healthcare efforts. Even so, many difficult lessons were learned that health professionals apply today.

Providing emergency medical care to mass casualty survivors requires healthcare professionals to solve problems very quickly. In 2013, two bombs exploded at the Boston Marathon, sending hundreds of injured people to 27 hospitals in the Boston area. The quick adaptation of hospital procedures by the medical staff, including the radiologists, and their activating their EOP, facilitated the diagnosis and treatment of seriously injured patients.

As described in the EVD case, when serious threats are posed by infectious disease agents, healthcare systems have to isolate patients, quickly analyze appropriate specimens, provide a diagnosis and treatment, trace contacts, and communicate effectively to the staff and the public to prevent further outbreaks. In 2014, the first case of EVD was diagnosed in the US. The preparatory actions of the state laboratory in Texas allowed swift, accurate, and coordinated testing to occur for diagnosis and appropriate response. All cases provide lessons which hospitals can use to ensure that their EOPS address the types of issues that they may confront during emergencies and disasters.

Additional Resources

To extend the content presented in this chapter, take advantage of the resources available through the chapter's eBook resource links and the end-of-chapter link. These resources include informational supplements and flash cards for terms and abbreviations.

Key Terms	
access and functional needs	medical surge
assay	memorandum of understanding
biosafety protocols	national laboratory
Biothreat Team	personal protective equipment
blast injuries	presumptive result
casualty collection point	reagent
computed tomography (CT)	reference laboratory
contact tracing	select agent
credentials	sentinel laboratory
Emergency Use Authorization	staging area
evacuation	The Joint Commission
external quality assurance review	triple packaging
index patient	unidentified patient naming convention
job action sheet	

Recognizing Terms

Choose the word or phrase from the list of key terms that best matches each of the following descriptions. Your instructor may ask you to submit your work for grading or may provide you with an answer key for self-assessment.

1. Place at the scene of an incident where medical personnel bring patients, to assess, and stabilize their medical conditions, and then send them to hospitals for care ________
2. The national organization that conducts accreditation of health facilities ________
3. A substance that has the potential to pose a severe threat to public health and safety ________
4. Injuries from explosions ________
5. Proof of education and professional skills ________
6. How to give a name to a patient whose identity is not known ________
7. Having difficulty taking care of oneself or understanding the implications of what may be happening ________

8. The type of packaging required for the transport of highly infectious biological specimens __________
9. Safety procedures for handling highly infectious biological materials __________
10. Gowns, goggles, gloves, masks, and special respiratory protection worn to reduce exposure to highly infectious diseases __________

Reviewing Concepts

Choose the response that best answers the question or completes the sentence. Your instructor may ask you to submit your work for grading or may provide you with an answer key for self-assessment.

1. How often should healthcare facilities conduct emergency preparedness drills?
   a. monthly
   b. once a year
   c. twice a year
   d. every other year
2. Why is it important that healthcare facilities stay open after a disaster?
   a. Patients don't want to reschedule appointments.
   b. Staff need the income from their salary.
   c. Hospitals might lose their accreditation if they don't stay open.
   d. Patients with chronic diseases may get sicker if they cannot continue their care.
3. What should be done to preserve vaccines during a disaster?
   a. Pack them in ice.
   b. Be sure that there is a generator with fuel to provide backup power.
   c. Give them to the hospital for safekeeping.
   d. Take them home.
4. What are the types of damages that can occur to a medical facility during a disaster? (chose all the answers that are correct)
   a. They lose power.
   b. Every patient wants to go home.
   c. Staff have difficulty getting to work.
   d. They run out of supplies.

5. Which of the following is *not* likely a problem that healthcare facilities experience after a disaster?
   a. staff shortages
   b. supply shortages
   c. uninterrupted communication
   d. fewer patients than usual seeking care
6. Why did hospitals have difficulty evacuating during Hurricane Katrina and after?
   a. It was too hard to fit people in the elevators.
   b. There were not enough staff to carry people down the stairs.
   c. The roads were flooded, and the buses and ambulances couldn't get to the hospitals.
   d. People refused to leave the hospitals.
7. Which of these was the least reliable solution for the loss of medical records after Hurricane Katrina?
   a. A website was created that allowed doctors to see a patient's medical history and a list of their medications.
   b. Doctors depended on patient's families to provide medical information.
   c. Some health information professionals backed up records on laptop computers, flash drives, or handheld devices.
   d. Health professionals created medical summaries on paper, and these were transported with patients.
8. Why is it important to transport a patient with his or her wheelchair?
   a. Wheelchairs can easily be replaced.
   b. A wheelchair may be customized for the person who uses it.
   c. Someone else will bring the wheelchair to the person.
   d. It is easy to identify which wheelchair belongs to which person.
9. Why did most victims of the Boston Marathon bombing survive?
   a. Teams of medical staff were located near the site of the explosion, and they used tourniquets to control bleeding.
   b. Most people did not have serious injuries.
   c. The hospitals in Boston that can care for trauma patients were located close by.
   d. There were enough ambulances to transport everyone to the hospital.

10. Why did the radiology technicians have difficulty taking the necessary X-rays following the Boston Marathon bombing?
    a. There were not enough portable X-ray machines.
    b. They needed special training.
    c. The patients needed to go to surgery immediately after arrival.
    d. There was no power to run the machines.

11. Why was there confusion about which tests were ordered following the Boston Marathon bombing?
    a. The physicians were all trying to order the tests at the same time.
    b. The system couldn't process so many requests.
    c. The medical staff did not know who the patients were when they arrived and did not have a good unidentified patient naming convention.
    d. The order system was not working.

12. What is an Emergency Use Authorization?
    a. an order by a health commissioner to use a special procedure in an emergency
    b. an FDA action which allows the special use of a medical product to diagnose or treat serious life-threatening diseases when there are no available alternatives
    c. the use of lifesaving drugs in the emergency department
    d. permission by the LEMA to use equipment and supplies stored for emergencies

13. The most specialized laboratories in the Laboratory Response Network are the
    a. sentinel laboratories.
    b. reference laboratories.
    c. national laboratories.
    d. international laboratories.

14. What did the laboratory in Austin do to determine it it was ready to test the Ebola specimen?
    a. Review the location of the lab.
    b. Wash down the walls and equipment.
    c. Make sure everyone had a personal disaster plan.
    d. Make sure it had the correct biosafety protocols.

15. Which healthcare facilities had the most difficulty in the days following Hurricane Katrina?
    a. those where normal operations could continue
    b. those that did not evacuate
    c. those that had a plan to call staff in
    d. those that were located away from where the storm hit
    e. those that had a disaster plan in place

Exploring Emergency Preparedness Issues

Complete the following activities to further explore the concepts found in this chapter. Your instructor may ask you to submit your work for grading or may provide you with guidance for self-assessment.

1. Visit your local hospital and ask if you can volunteer for its next disaster exercise.
2. Search for disasters that occurred in your state using the following website: **http://EmDPrp2.ParadigmEducation.com/DisastersByState.**

   Check with the local newspaper to find out if the disasters damaged any healthcare systems and what was done to respond and recover.
3. To learn about the CDC's role in responding to EVD, go to **http://EmDPrp2.ParadigmEducation.com/CDCEbola.**
4. Considering what you have learned, what should your community do to get ready for the next emerging infectious disease?

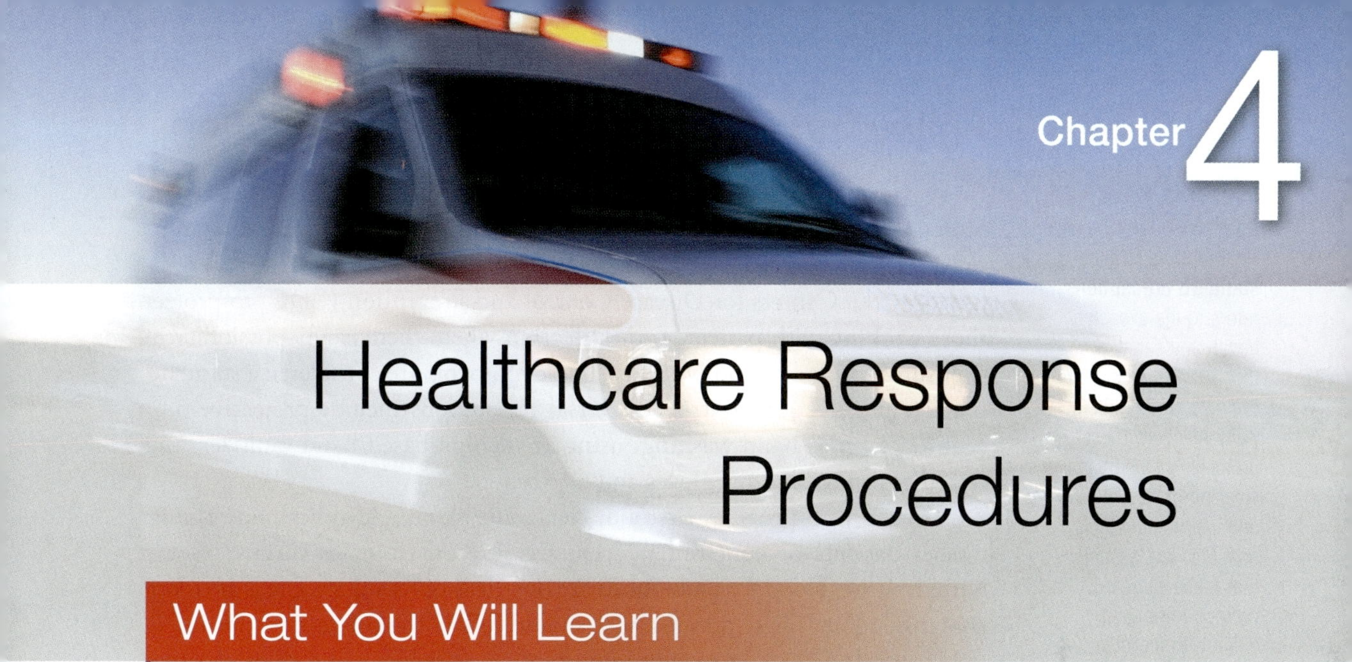

Chapter 4

Healthcare Response Procedures

What You Will Learn

- How to protect yourself and patients with universal and standard precautions
- How to protect yourself through wearing personal protective equipment
- What triage is and how it is conducted
- How to triage patients after a chemical, biological, radiological, or nuclear disaster
- How the Laboratory Response Network investigates infectious diseases or suspicious specimens
- How to control disease through social distancing methods
- How to communicate risks to the public and patients
- The setup and staffing of a Point of Dispensing site and how the federal stockpiles of medications and supplies are distributed
- How to to prepare for and communicate the reopening of a health facility after a disaster

Emergency and disaster response involves a variety of special healthcare procedures, both at the initial response site and within the medical facility. For example, procedures exist for evaluating many patients at the same time and sending them to varying types of care, decontaminating patients, investigating suspicious specimens in the lab, and more. This chapter introduces you to the procedures that are common in emergency and disaster response.

Following Health and Safety Protocols

Expand Your Knowledge

Note that the term **standard precautions** refers to the expected health and safety protocols that protect both the patient and others from infection. These protocols include hand washing gloves, masks, and instrument sterilization. This text assumes that these standard protocols are used along with universal precautions.

Every day, regardless of whether an emergency or disaster occurs, healthcare professionals are expected to follow health and safety protocols known as universal precautions. **Universal precautions** are specific procedures established by the Centers for Disease Control and Prevention (CDC) to protect those working with patients from infection where there is any possibility of exposure to blood or bodily fluids. These protocols are considered a standard practice of infection control. Universal precautions include protective procedures, such as hand washing, using an alcohol-based hand sanitizer, and wearing disposable latex gloves and face masks.

Anyone who provides first aid; cleans up blood and other body fluids; washes patients or contaminated laundry; decontaminates surfaces where human tissue, blood, or body fluids are handled; or handles waste is at risk of contamination. These persons, too, should follow the precautions for infection control. This is especially important in emergency and disaster situations where typical routines and resources have been adversely affected. In an emergency or disaster, healthcare professionals will not know whether a patient they encounter has an infectious disease, such as HIV or hepatitis A, B, or C. Healthcare professionals should always assume that all body fluids they encounter are potentially infectious materials.

Be Aware

Alcohol-based hand sanitizers kill bacteria but are less effective if wiped off before they completely dry, or if the user does not use enough for the hands to be completely covered with the sanitizer.

Healthcare professionals responding to an emergency or disaster are expected to follow universal precautions and standard precautions, using sterile supplies and instruments to prevent the transmission of infectious diseases. If water and power are not available because of damage to facilities, other methods must be used, such as applying isopropyl alcohol to hands. In addition to universal precautions, additional protective equipment is also available for incidents where responders could be exposed to hazardous conditions.

Together, protective equipment and universal precautions protect responders and other healthcare workers from getting infected through contact with potentially infectious material.

Key Acronyms	
OSHA	Occupational Safety and Health Administration
POD	Point of Dispensing
START	simple triage and rapid treatment
SNS	Strategic National Stockpile

A Closer Look

Hand Washing without Water

All healthcare professionals know the importance of washing their hands often and correctly to stop the spread of infection. This simple task becomes even more important in emergencies that involve the possibility of infection or contaminants. However, after some emergencies such as a hurricane or flood, water supplies may be temporarily cut off or contaminated.

If soap and water are not available, alcohol-based hand sanitizers with a minimum of 60% alcohol can reduce the bacteria on the skin.

Sanitizing can be more effective in killing bacteria and viruses than soap and water in most situations, but not if the skin is dirty, because dirt keeps the sanitizer from reaching the skin.

Personal Protective Equipment

Before entering any emergency or disaster site, healthcare responders need to be prepared to protect themselves from injury. That is why first responders are highly trained in both infection control and safety protocols and in the use of safety equipment. All allied health professionals must be protected before responding in the field or at the emergency department of a hospital. They should receive direction as to their expected roles and the use of any personal protective equipment (PPE) needed to safely participate in the response. PPE is required by the **Occupational Safety and Health Administration (OSHA)**, which has oversight for workplace safety.

Once they understand how PPE will be used, each responder must be provided with the appropriate PPE. As discussed in Chapter 3, PPE includes gowns, goggles, gloves, masks, and special respiratory protection. Equipment that provides additional protection is required when more protection is needed.

The four levels of PPE are A, B, C, and D, going from highest protection to lesser protection in decreasingly hazardous situations.

- **Level A** includes a protective suit that covers every part of the body, protective long underwear, and a self-sustaining protective unit for breathing that supplies oxygen. You have probably seen pictures of workers in "moon suits" responding to hazardous material incidents. These workers were wearing Level A PPE. All responders need special training to work safely and effectively after a chemical, biological, or radiation incident, which includes how to use Level A equipment.
- **Level B** offers a positive pressure face mask and self-contained breathing apparatus that supplies oxygen no specialized underwear. The PPE includes a hooded, chemical-resistant coveralls and boot covers, and double gloves.

Be Aware

Respirators remove contaminants from the air that is breathed in, filtering out chemicals and gases, or provide clean air from a safe source, such as an air tank. There are several different types of respirators. Some have a hood with a seal and a neck piece.

- **Level C** has a full or half mask with a **respirator**, which is an apparatus that cleans the air for breathing, along with chemical-resistant covers for clothing, double gloves, and boots.
- **Level D** is the uniform that you wear at work every day with additional protection, such as gowns, aprons, gloves, boots or shoes, safety glasses, and a surgical face mask.

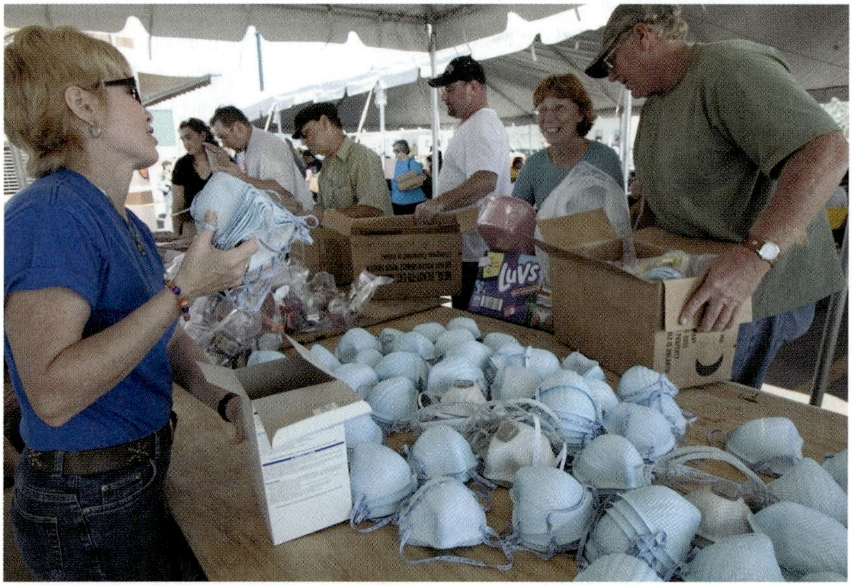

Volunteers are provided with proper personal protective equipment for helping with cleanup after Hurricane Katrina at the Chalmette Recovery Center in October 2005.

General Principles and Protocols of PPE

The appropriate type of clothing will depend on the task and degree of potential exposure. If patient care is likely to expose you to a splash or spray of blood or other body fluids, you will be instructed about what to wear and may receive additional training on how to **don and doff**, or put on and take off, the PPE. As noted, at a minimum as part of universal precautions, you will be directed to wear a clean, nonsterile gown, gloves, and a mask to protect your skin and prevent your clothing from being soiled. If possible, remove a soiled gown promptly and then wash your hands to prevent transfer of microorganisms.

During an emergency or disaster, the incident commander or team leader will determine the appropriate level of PPE needed for those under his or her direction. At hospital EDs, the emergency room physician, attending physician, or head nurse will use the notes from the first responders or medical record information along with symptoms to determine if additional PPE is needed beyond Level D.

Additional Hand Protection If you are in a situation in which you may be exposed to harmful substances, extreme temperatures that could cause burns, or sharp objects that could cause cuts, abrasions, or punctures, you will be directed to protect your hands with a heavy-duty type of glove or double gloves. Change gloves after you touch material that may contain a high concentration of microorganisms or chemicals. Remove gloves promptly after using them, before touching uncontaminated items or caring for another patient.

Eye and Face Protection Wear face shields and goggles whenever there is a potential for flying particles, molten metal, acids or other caustic liquids, or gases. Wearing gear that protects the eyes and face is essential in the aftermath of explosions, during search and rescue, and at fires.

Emergency eyewash facilities should be provided in all areas where eyes may be exposed to potentially dangerous materials, such as in a fire, explosion, or chemical release.

Medical Mask Medical masks protect against harmful substances in the air, such as smoke and chemicals, or infectious agents. When examining or treating patients with symptoms of a respiratory infection, masks are needed, particularly if fever is present. They also remind people not to touch their faces. Change a mask when it becomes moist, and do not leave a mask dangling around your neck.

Be Aware

"N95" indicates that the mask can filter out particles down to 0.3 microns, which includes viruses, 95% of the time if properly fit tested.

If a mask is not available at an incident site, cover your nose and mouth with several layers of a cotton T-shirt or towel or scarf, or use several layers of tissue or paper towels. A regular medical mask does not provide protection from viruses. Viruses are too small to be caught by the fibers of a mask. To be

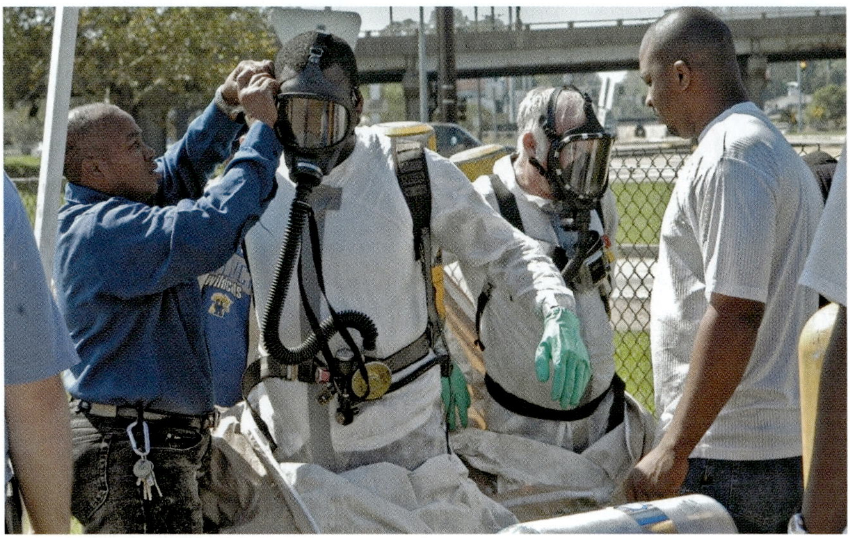

In a simulation exercise for cleaning up a chemical spill in Baton Rouge, Louisiana, an emergency responder is being fit tested for his respirator, and the HAZMAT instructor is adjusting it to fit correctly. (See "A Closer Look" on the next page.)

protected against viruses, healthcare professionals need to wear a specialized respirator mask, the N95 respirator.

Respirators The respirators needed for Level C protection are designed to prevent the inhalation of very small particles, such as viruses, harmful dust, fumes, vapors, or gases. This level of respiratory protection (or higher) is required when airborne contaminants at a disaster site exceed a certain level established by OSHA.

A Closer Look

Fit Testing Masks and Respirators

Before using an N95 mask or respirator, a person must be **fit tested**, or specifically fitted and tested, for the proper make, model, style, and size. Fit testing must be done whenever a different respirator is worn and must be redone at least once a year. Workers also must pass classroom and on-site training before using a respirator.

In April 2003, hospital staff learned the importance of using the correct level of facial protection. It took only a few hours for nine Canadian first responders and healthcare workers in Toronto to contract severe acute respiratory syndrome (SARS) after caring for an infected patient. Six were exposed because they were in the room when a tube was placed into the windpipe of the patient to help him breathe. The droplets forced from the patient's mouth contained a high concentration of the SARS virus. An investigation revealed that the healthcare workers were wearing protective gear including gloves, googles, and surgical masks. However, the healthcare personnel would have been better protected if they had worn N-95 respirators that had been fit tested, as the medical masks did not provide the protection required and air infected with the SARS virus was able to enter under the medical mask.

Mass Casualty Triage

Now that you know what protection equipment and infection-control protocols are required to protect yourself, you will be ready to help with the medical response at the scene of the incident and in the healthcare facility. When many people have been injured at one time, healthcare providers need to rapidly identify which people need immediate treatment, which are most likely to survive, and which can benefit the most from treatment.

For instance, imagine that a train collides with a car stalled on the train tracks in your community. The train jackknifes, and many people are injured. First responders (EMS, fire, and police) will race to the scene.

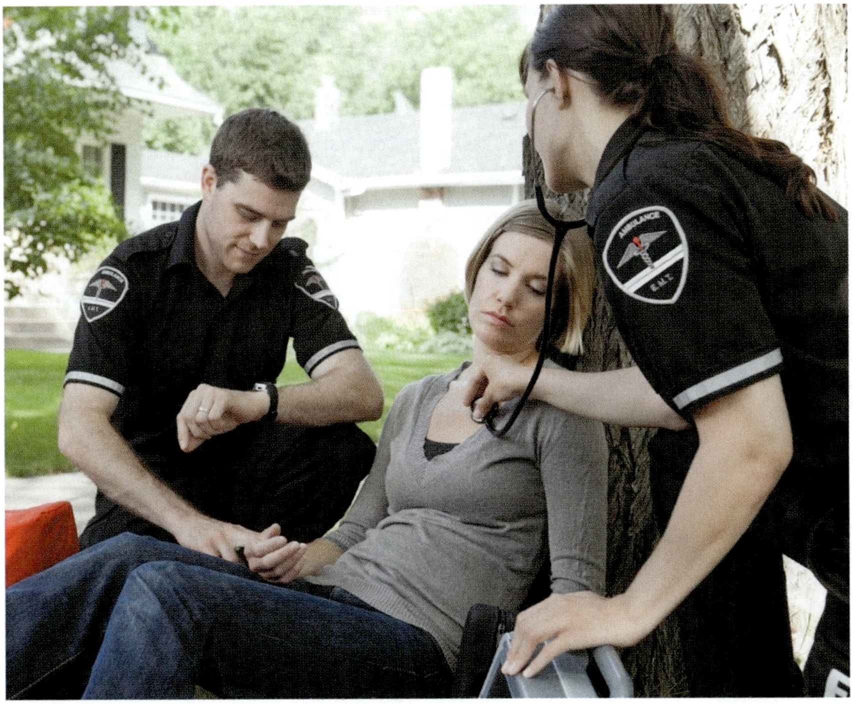

Responders check a patient's vital signs. Paramedics and emergency medical technicans (EMTs) are the allied health professionals best qualified for on-site triage.

The incident commander and first responders will set up or clear an area where they will assess the injured and sort them into groups for treatment and transport. Only the most basic lifesaving treatments will be provided on the scene, and those victims with hope for survival will be transported to a treatment center. Some injured will be transported by ambulance to the nearest hospitals with emergency departments (EDs). The most seriously injured will be sent to the closest level 1 trauma center. If patients have died, they will be delivered to a nearby on-site morgue for transport to a regular morgue, where their loved ones will be notified.

The procedure for sorting victims according to their conditions, treatment needs, and available resources is called **triage**. During triage, the responders check a patient's vital signs and obvious life-threatening injuries. They assess the patient's condition and attach a triage tag. Everyone who cares for the injured after triage will take appropriate actions based on the color of the triage tags. (More will be explained about the tags in a section to come.)

Paramedics and emergency medical technicians (EMTs) are the allied health professionals best qualified and most likely to participate in on-site triage. As described, they do not begin treatment during triage except to provide immediate lifesaving care, such as opening an air passageway or applying tourniquets to stop life-threatening bleeding.

Be Aware

Healthcare facilities with trauma centers are ranked from 1, with comprehensive services, to 3, with limited services, by the American College of Surgeons.

In June, 2016, students in a program at the Center for Domestic Preparedness practice triage techniques in a simulated emergency on a bus or subway.

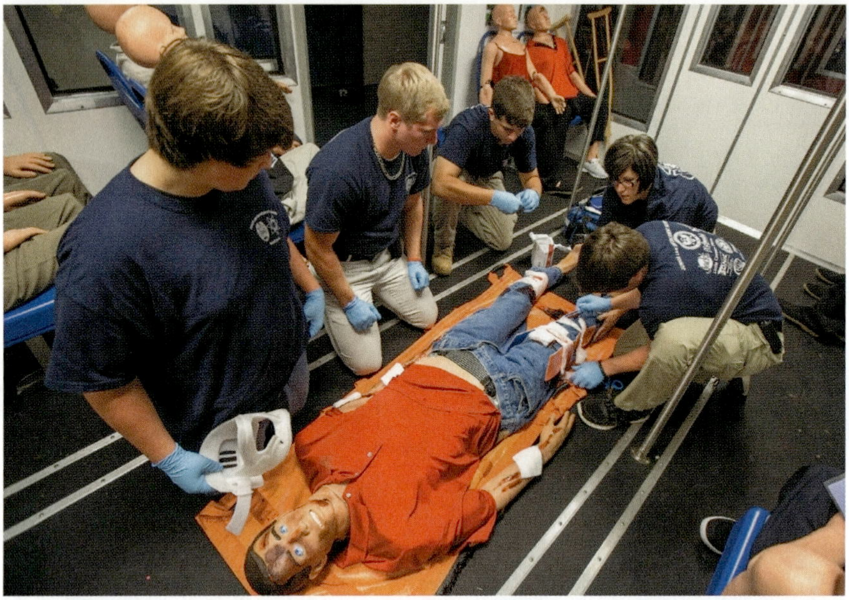

After establishing the site for triage, the on-site triage team works to accomplish the following goals:

- Estimate how many patients need to be evaluated to alert the EMS dispatchers
- Estimate how many ambulances are needed
- Evaluate and tag patients
- Transport patients to the ambulance loading area and prepare them for transport to hospitals

Triage is not limited to the emergency or disaster site. For example, if a building collapses, triage would begin at the site, but a second triage at the hospital may also be necessary because the patients' conditions may have changed by the time they reach the ED. Also, the ED is likely to be receiving many patients at once, not only those triaged at the incident site, but also those who could transport themselves to the hospital and those who are part of the normal flow of ED patients. The ED may need to triage patients to decide who gets treated first based on their condition. In anticipation of the arrival of many patients at once, based on the dispatcher's information, the ED may need to call in additional staff from other parts of the hospital to assist. In the ED, the triage teams are generally led by an emergency physician or trauma specialist. Allied health professionals may be assigned to a triage team to provide support functions.

Triage may also be performed in other medical settings. For example, on September 11, 2001, thousands of people who were caught in the dust and debris from the collapse of the World Trade Center sought medical treatment at hospitals outside the immediate region and at offices of private doctors throughout the New York metropolitan area. Triage occurred in almost every setting where victims arrived.

Simple Triage and Rapid Treatment Tagging

In most mass casualty incidents, experience has shown that about one-third of the patients will be critically injured and two-thirds will be noncritical. However, when a building collapses or explodes, the proportions change, and many more people could be critically injured.

With injured patients, the triage process cannot take long. Most injured people can be triaged in one minute or less. This means two people conducting triage can handle 20 patients in 10 minutes. Several well-established methods are used to triage patients in the field. Different communities may use different systems for different types of emergencies.

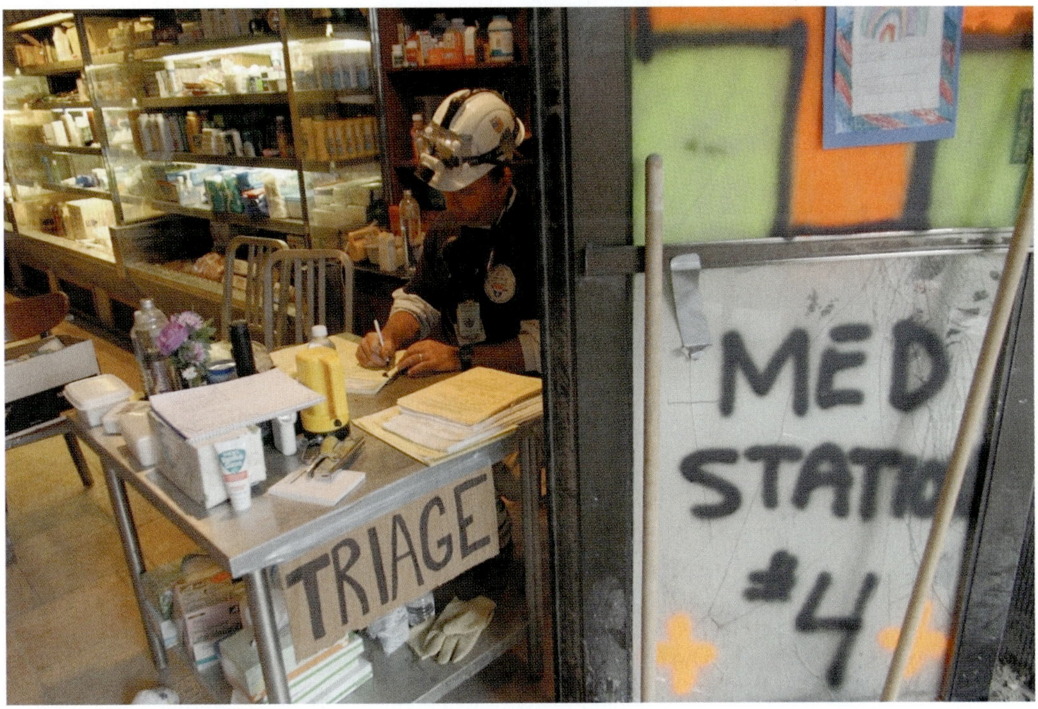

Amidst the trauma and confusion of September 11, first responders risked their lives (and many lost them), seeking to save and tend to others. Medical triage stations were set up ad hoc wherever there was a safe space. This medical station was established in a New York City store and was still open six days later for anyone needing medical evaluation and direction.

An effective method of triage is **Simple Triage And Rapid Treatment (START)**. START makes it possible for only a few rescuers, even those with limited training, to rapidly triage many patients and move them to treatment centers for more detailed assessment. The START system separates mass casualty patients into four clinical categories, each with its own color code: red for those needing immediate care, yellow for those who can have delayed care, green for those mobile enough to walk away to receive care, and black for those unlikely to survive or already dead. Those conducting triage follow clinical guidelines to evaluate each patient. They assess such factors as:

- Ability to walk away from the scene
- Presence or absence of spontaneous breathing
- Respiratory rate greater or less than 30 per minute
- Pulse rate between 60 and 100 beats per minute
- Mental status assessed by the ability of the patient to respond to commands

A Closer Look

START Triage System

The four categories that physicians and allied health personnel sort patients into with the START triage system are the following:

Immediate—Red Triage Tag

- Victim can be helped if immediate care and transport is received.
- Requires medical attention within 60 minutes to survive.
- Patient's airway, breathing, and circulation are compromised. For example, patient's condition is critical and life-threatening, such as when the patient is hemorrhaging or in shock.

Delayed—Yellow Triage Tag

- Transport of the victim can be delayed.
- Victim has serious and life-threatening injuries, but status is not expected to deteriorate significantly in the next several hours. For example, patients may have an open fracture or chest wound.

Walking Wounded—Green Triage Tag

- Victim has relatively minor injuries and is able to move on his or her own out of the incident site to a treatment area. Examples include closed fracture, sprain, or strain.
- Status is unlikely to deteriorate.
- Victim may be able to assist in his or her own care.

Deceased or Expectant—Black Triage Tag

- Victim is dead or unlikely to survive, given the severity of injuries, level of available care, or both. Examples include massive head injury or extensive burns.
- Victim should be made as comfortable as possible, and pain relief should be provided.

Ethical Dilemmas in Triage

People who do not understand the principles and goals of the life-and-death decisions in triage may find it difficult both ethically and emotionally to participate. Although the goal of everyday healthcare is to provide the best possible care to every patient, in an incident involving many injured people, the goal is to provide the best possible care to those patients who are most likely to survive. These decisions must be made swiftly, based on the available resources at the scene.

For example, if many people need a ventilator to survive and the number of ventilators is insufficient, those conducting triage will decide who receives a ventilator and who does not. Those who are not expected to live would not be placed on ventilators. These decisions would be made to avoid diverting scarce resources away from patients more likely to survive.

Since this is a difficult paradigm in healthcare, learning about the reasons for triage will help you be more comfortable and effective if you are called on to help.

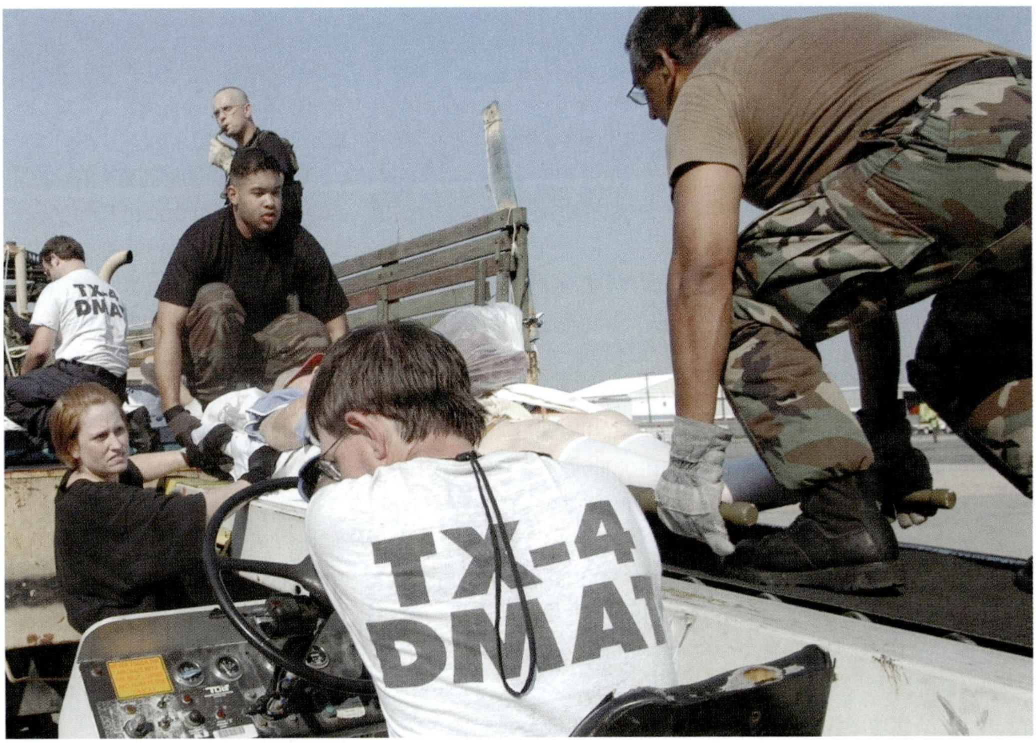

In the stifling heat, members of the Texas-4 DMAT and the Louisiana National Guard use litters to carry patients evacuated from dangerous areas of New Orleans to a triage area in the aftermath of Hurricane Katrina.

Allied Health Professionals Supporting Triage Teams

Allied health professionals can function in specific or supporting roles in triage. For example, respiratory therapists and technicians can assess opening airways during triage or provide ventilator or other respiratory care at the hospital.

They may also assist in transporting patients to waiting ambulances or nearby treatment areas. This requires specific equipment, such as stretchers. The people who move the victims are known as **litter bearers**; they are formed into teams of three or four people and report to the triage unit leader for their assignments. The litter bearers transport patients to the designated area where patients are loaded into the ambulances.

A Closer Look

Reporting Human Remains

When triage is performed at a site, uninjured family members and friends are asked to stay clear of the area to let the emergency responders work, just as at a hospital. If victims die in triage, they are tagged with black tags and transported last. If loved ones are nearby waiting, there are protocols for handling this. Different incident commanders or Local Emergency Management Agencies (LEMAs) have different guidelines for handling this. If you are working at a site, it is important to know the protocols.

When you are assisting in providing care or volunteering to help in cleanup at an emergency or disaster site, you may also encounter victims who have died. Victims of natural disasters often die from drowning or trauma and are not likely to have an infection. However, because of the possible presence of infectious diseases, bodies should be handled only by workers who have special training and equipment, including a powered air-purifying respirator.

If you are on-site and encounter a body, notify someone from public safety. Trained workers will place the body in a body bag, attach a tag with any known information, and release it to the medical examiner. It is important that all human remains are handled with respect and dignity.

The goals of triage are to save all who can be saved. For those who cannot be saved, it is essential that everything is done to preserve the evidence and information about where the body was found, so that the person can be properly identified and the remains can be united with loved ones.

Triage after Exposure to Chemical, Biological, Radiological, and Nuclear Agents

Triaging patients in incidents that involve exposure to chemical, biological, radiological, or nuclear (CBRN) agents requires additional special procedures and protection that differ from other mass casualty incidents. Contamination occurs when a person, surface, or object comes into direct contact with the toxic substance or with something that has it on or in it.

This can occur in an explosion, leak, emission, contact with a contaminated item, or encounter with an infected person. **Contaminated patients** are those who have been exposed to a CBRN substance on their clothes and/or in or on their bodies.

To handle a CBRN incident, highly trained responders conduct the triage of contaminated patients in three locations:

- **Hot zone:** This is the area immediately next to where the victim was exposed to the hazardous material. All healthcare personnel wear the highest level of PPE. Minimal treatment occurs in the hot zone except to help people whose airways are compromised, who are bleeding, or who require **antidotes**—substances that can counteract a form of disease or poison that they were exposed to. Triage in this zone is generally very simple, between those patients who are able to walk (ambulatory) to the next zone and those who are not.
- **Warm zone:** This area, at least 300 feet away and upwind and uphill from the incident, is set up for the decontamination of patients. **Decontamination** is the removal or neutralization of harmful substances, such as chemical agents or radioactive materials. Such substances can penetrate clothing and are absorbed rapidly through the skin. Patients are rapidly sorted into traditional triage treatment categories. Those who are not ambulatory will go through a decontamination process while they lie on stretchers. Victims who can walk go through ambulatory decontamination.

Contamination – Decontamination Control Zones

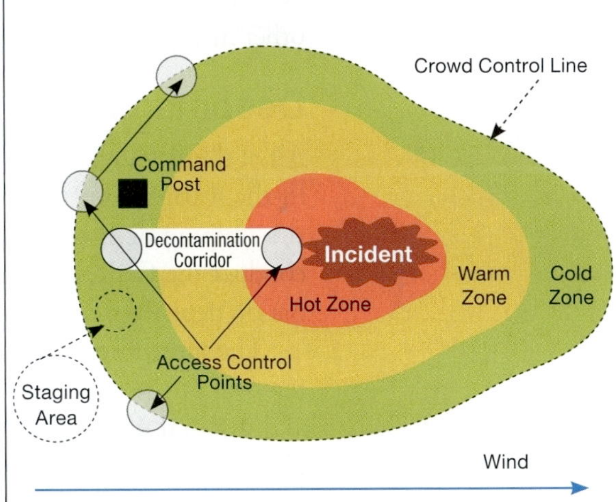

Be Aware

The term **ambulatory** indicates that a patient can walk without assistance.

- **Cold zone:** This is an area next to the warm zone that is far enough away from the incident area and the decontamination processes to be free of contamination. Here the decontaminated patients are sorted for transport to the proper facility. In this zone, responders may continue to wear PPE in case the wind changes or victims were improperly decontaminated.

CBRN Triage Procedures

The CBRN triage involves sorting patients into the following three categories:

- Individuals most seriously harmed from exposure, as with burns, and needing immediate treatment
- Individuals in need of treatment such as a chemical antidote or an antibiotic to prevent infection
- Individuals who do not need medical care because they have died, been immunized, or have recovered enough to be discharged

Those with the most severe symptoms are treated first. Patients are also evaluated for secondary injuries and sent for treatment for exposure and other medical needs.

Decontamination Procedures

All of those who have been exposed go through the decontamination process in the warm zone. The most effective decontamination is done within the first minute or two after someone is exposed. Specially trained responders conduct the CBRN decontamination. The level and method of decontamination depends on the type of incident.

The most important part of decontamination is the timely and effective removal of the contaminant from the patient. The first step is the removal and disposal of clothing. Clothing and contaminated belongings should be placed in a sealed vapor-resistant bag that will be disposed of as part of hazardous waste.

Victims must then shower or be showered with plenty of warm water and a hypoallergenic liquid soap. This is followed by more warm water and then a final rinse. Sponges and disposable towels are used and then disposed of along with the clothing. The decontamination tent or facility should provide gowns or other temporary clothing.

If healthcare professionals are asked to help with the decontamination of patients, they would be given an initial briefing on PPE, the hazard, and their duties.

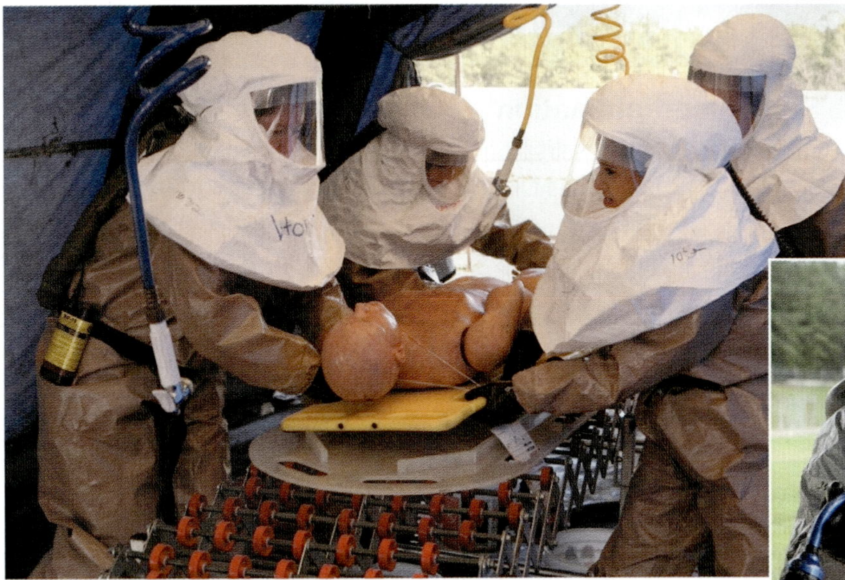

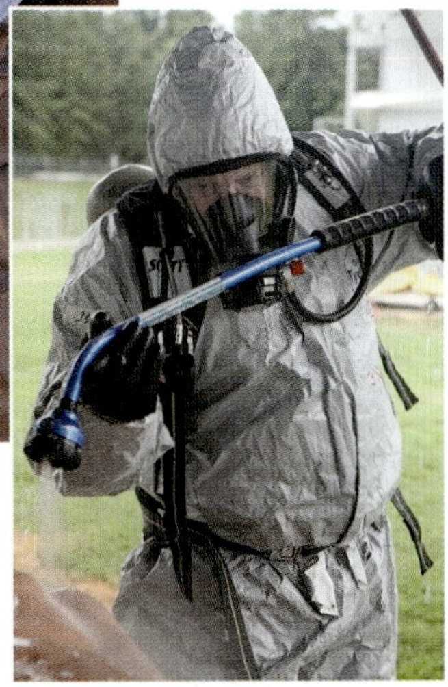

In a simulation of an incident involving chemical exposure, healthcare workers swiftly decontaminate the "victim". These students at the Center for Domestic Preparedness participated in the Hospital Emergency Response Training for Mass Casualty Incidents course. The instructor shows how to decontaminate a patient.

Many hospitals depend on the local fire department to handle decontamination before patients get to the hospital. If a CBRN event is large, the fire department may not be able to help at the hospital. Therefore, designated hospitals prepare to conduct their own decontamination of patients. They must set up hot, warm, and cold zones on their site. Some facilities use their parking lots to set up tent facilities for some of these zones. The facility conducting the decontamination should provide the following:

- Climate-controlled shelter
- Separate areas for men and women so that they can remove contaminated clothing with some privacy
- Separate areas for washing off the chemical agent
- A method for containing and disposing of contaminated wastewater
- A place for dumping the contaminated clothing and bandages
- A temporary morgue for deceased patients

Despite protective steps, some hazardous substances may still expose health professionals to risk. In 1995, terrorists released the nerve agent sarin on the Tokyo subway. Hospital personnel were initially misinformed that a gas explosion had caused burns and carbon monoxide poisoning. When

A Closer Look

Self-Decontamination

To decontaminate yourself, act quickly and follow the instructions you are given. You will probably be told to:

- Quickly take off all clothing that may have any contaminant on it. Cut off any clothing that must be pulled over your head.
- Place your clothing inside a vapor-resistant plastic bag. Anything that touched the contaminated clothing should also be placed in the bag.
- As quickly as possible, wash any contaminant from your skin, using large amounts of soap and water.
- If your eyes are burning or your vision is blurred, rinse your eyes with plain water for 10 to 15 minutes.
- Remove contact lenses and discard them with your contaminated clothing. Do not put the contact lenses back in your eyes. Eyeglasses can be washed with soap and water and put back on.
- Avoid contact with people who may have been exposed to contaminants, but who have not yet changed their clothes or washed.
- Move away from the area where the chemical or infectious agent was released.
- Report the location of the bags where you deposited your contaminated items, but do not move them yourself.

patients arrived in great numbers to the main receiving hospital, hospital staff members had the patients shower. The patients' clothing was placed in plastic bags and sealed. Staff members used surgical masks and gloves. However, three hours after the release, hospital staff learned that the victims had been exposed to sarin. Despite the protective steps taken, more than 100 hospital staff members (23%) experienced acute poisoning symptoms.

Emergency Response in Medical Laboratories

In incidents involving CBRN substances or infectious diseases, accurate laboratory findings are crucial for determining the right medical treatment for the patients and the best strategy for protecting the public. If patients have been exposed to a toxic chemical, it is important to quickly identify the type of chemical to be able to neutralize or treat it with the proper antidote.

After public exposure to CBRN substances or infectious diseases, hospital medical laboratories will likely have more samples than normal to test. The tests may require more complex sets of procedures than usual. When the hospital physicians or local public health authorities suspect that a material is suspicious or an agent is highly infectious, a sample will be sent to a reference lab in the Laboratory Response Network (LRN) to identity and analyze it.

Laboratory Emergency Response Guidelines

The LRN provides guidelines to medical laboratories in healthcare facilities around the nation on how to respond when they receive suspicious specimens. Some key rules include the following:

A sentinel lab should never accept a sample that is suspected of being a bioterrorist agent. Such specimens should be sent directly to the nearest reference laboratory.

If a lab test is being conducted and a possible bioterrorism agent is grown in the lab or detected in any other way, the lab staff should immediately

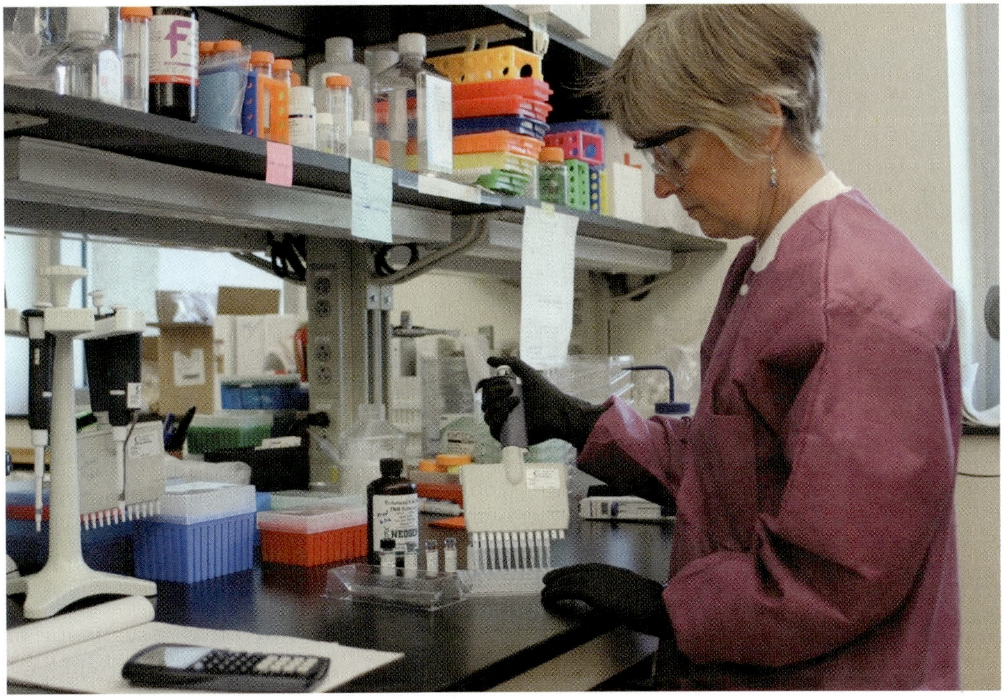

At the Division of Vector-Borne Diseases in Fort Collins, CO, a microbiologist prepares the reagent for the test to determine the presence of the Zika virus.

Expand Your Knowledge

Every lab has procedures for processing suspicious specimens. These procedures are based on guidelines from the LRN and other professional organizations, such as the Infectious Diseases Society of America and the American Society for Microbiology. To learn more, go to: http://EmDPrp2.ParadigmEducation.com/suspicious-specimens.

notify the lab supervisor and anyone else listed in the lab's emergency plan, such as the treating physician. The supervisor or lab manager will likely be designated in the plan to contact the director and infection control officer as well as state and local health departments.

A supervisor at a sentinel lab should contact a reference lab for instructions about how to handle a suspicious agent before sending it to another lab for confirmation.

In addition to collecting the test samples, the medical lab at the healthcare facility is responsible for properly handling and shipping clinical samples. The specimens may also be needed as evidence in a criminal or Federal Bureau of Investigation (FBI) investigation.

Communicating Lab Results to Agencies and Healthcare Facilities

While doing their work, laboratories that are part of the LRN must coordinate with many agencies, such as state DOH authorities, law enforcement, and emergency management authorities. When a national lab confirms that a specimen is a biological or chemical agent, it notifies the CDC, FBI, state emergency management authorities, and state or local public health officials, who contact the reporting healthcare facility. If authorities believe that a biological substance was released as an act of terrorism, both a criminal and a public health investigation will be initiated. The state and county health departments and the CDC will work with the healthcare facility to deliver the proper treatment to the infected and exposed patients and their healthcare team. As explained in Chapter 3, a public health investigation and contact tracing will determine how many people were exposed. All this can happen within hours of identifying the specimen.

Controlling Infectious Disease Exposure

As noted in Chapter 1, people known to be infected or exposed to a highly infectious disease need to be kept separate from those who are healthy or unexposed to keep the infection from spreading. It is important that patients who may have an infectious disease be identified as soon as possible. Most healthcare facilities screen patients upon arrival for fever, respiratory symptoms, and rashes. Healthcare facilities have standard operating procedures specifically for the management of patients with different symptoms of infectious diseases, called **infection control procedures**. A facility will have one set of protocols for symptoms of fever and rash, another set for fever and respiratory symptoms, and so on.

For highly infectious diseases, health professionals use **social distancing** techniques, where distance or a barrier is established between affected individuals and others. The goal of social distancing is to decrease the number of people who are exposed to a potentially infectious disease to reduce its transmission. Hospitals follow the county or state health department rules for using social distancing methods based on state laws (which vary from state to state). There are two types of social distancing actions: isolation and quarantine.

Isolation is used to separate healthy people from those who are sick with an infectious disease. Isolation is part of daily practice in all healthcare settings. Infected patients can also be cared for in their own homes. The sick person is kept away from those who are not sick for as long as the disease can be transmitted from the patient to other people, which varies by disease. For example, someone with tuberculosis will be put in a single room separated from other patients. The people caring for him or her need to wear PPE. In emergency and disaster response to a serious outbreak, epidemic, or pandemic, isolation procedures can be implemented on a broader or more urgent scale in the case of an emerging infectious disease.

Quarantine is used to separate people who have been exposed to an infectious disease and may be infected but are not yet ill, from people who have not been exposed. The exposed individuals may still become infectious or be carriers and spread the disease to others.

Quarantine includes restricting the local movement and travel of individuals who have been exposed to an infectious disease. One example is a nurse who had a fever after returning from treating Ebola patients in Africa in 2014. The governor declared a state public health emergency and mandated that the nurse be quarantined until it could be determined whether she had Ebola Virus Disease.

Quarantined individuals can be monitored in a hospital or at home, depending on the disease, available resources, and regulations in that state or area. If it is a federally designated infectious disease, the federal government may try to enforce quarantines. Quarantined individuals receive all available medical interventions to prevent and control the infection. People are quarantined for as long as it takes for symptoms to develop after exposure.

The CDC recommends the least restrictive means of isolating or quarantining an individual to balance the protection of the public's health and an individual's civil rights. If exposed individuals are a threat to public health and are unwilling to be isolated or quarantined, they may legally be forced to comply. In an emergency, the state health department may order a required implementation of isolation and quarantine. The CDC must provide translation services when needed during the medical review and when issuing federal orders.

Expand Your Knowledge

For more information on the enforcement of patient isolation and quarantine, go to the CDC: **http://EmDPrp2.ParadigmEducation.com/quarantine.**

Web

Individuals who are detained or held in federal isolation or quarantine must receive adequate food and water, appropriate accommodation, appropriate medical treatment, and the tools to conduct necessary communication.

Care of Isolated or Quarantined Patients

Patients who require social distancing should be housed in rooms with separate ventilation systems. Some patients with similar symptoms for certain diseases can be grouped together as **cohorted patients**. (Those suspected of tuberculosis, however, would not be placed in a cohorted situation, as they may have different strains of the disease.) Privacy barriers, such as room dividers, should be used if possible to separate cohorted patients.

Equipment with patient contact, such as blood pressure cuffs and stethoscopes, should be left in the infected patient's room. This equipment should not be used on other patients unless it has been carefully cleaned and disinfected.

Patients are usually willing to be temporarily isolated or quarantined if their personal needs are met, including ways to pass the time. If necessary, arrangements should also be made to meet some of the needs of their families, since the person in isolation or quarantine cannot go to work.

A Closer Look

Diseases Requiring Isolation and Quarantine

The CDC can require isolation and quarantine for the following infectious diseases:

- Cholera
- Diphtheria
- Infectious tuberculosis
- Plague
- Smallpox
- Yellow fever
- Viral hemorrhagic fevers, such as EVD
- Severe acute respiratory syndrome
- Flu that can cause a pandemic

This list, current in May 2017, is subject to any executive order of the President to revise or add to it.

The CDC has the authority to detain anyone (regardless of citizenship or nationality) infected with one of the federally listed highly infectious diseases from traveling between states and into the US from other countries. The CDC has 72 hours from the time that an individual is detained to issue a federal order for isolation, quarantine, or conditional release. The list of diseases has been approved by the President, and the President can issue an executive order to revise or add a new disease to the list. For more information, go to: **http://EmDPrp2.ParadigmEducation.com/CSC-quarantine**.

Web

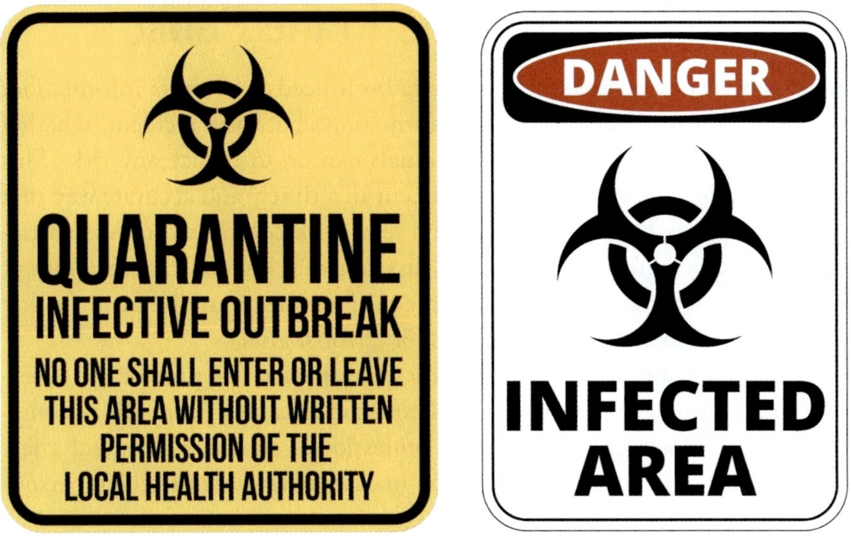
QUARANTINE
INFECTIVE OUTBREAK
NO ONE SHALL ENTER OR LEAVE THIS AREA WITHOUT WRITTEN PERMISSION OF THE LOCAL HEALTH AUTHORITY
DANGER
INFECTED AREA

The Secretary of the US Department of Health and Human Services (HHS) can establish, isolate, or quarantine when a highly infectious disease is suspected. A week after the September 11th attacks in 2001, anthrax spores were sent to several media outlets among others. Five people died from infection and 17 others were infected. Biohazard and quarantine signs similar to these were placed on the front door of the American Media building in Boca Raton, Florida.

When working with people who have been isolated or quarantined, it is critical that healthcare professionals consistently use universal precautions and the proper PPE. Some facilities require that healthcare professionals and family observe **droplet precautions**. Whenever family or healthcare professionals are within three feet of a patient, they need to don a face mask to prevent contact with microorganisms that may be transmitted in droplets. Healthcare professionals who handle patient linen or laundry should also use PPE when they are working in areas where patients have been isolated or quarantined.

In the event of an epidemic or pandemic, there may not be enough hospital space to care for all patients, and many patients will need to be treated at home. Communities have established the criteria for home isolation and quarantine in their pandemic preparedness plans. Families and caregivers should wear masks and gloves when caring for patients at home. The condition of each patient must be monitored. The patients or their families/caregivers may be asked to report by phone or via the Internet to a hospital, clinic, or medical provider's office. Health professionals from the county or state health department may be assigned to visit or contact patients for reports.

Communicating Risks to the Public

In an emergency or disaster, the public both needs and seeks information. **Risk communication** is relaying information about the incident, whether the public is at risk, and what individuals can do to reduce any risk. This kind of public communication must occur in a timely and accurate way that does not unduly heighten concern and fear. Risk communication is particularly important in emergencies and disasters that involve the possibility of additional threats, such as from the spread of an infectious disease or further earthquake tremors or weather events, or terrorist attacks.

Most often, a community or facility spokesperson will provide the necessary information. The designated spokesperson is usually the public information officer. However, all healthcare professionals should understand a few basic principles of risk communication in case patients talk to them personally about events. Individuals, outside agencies, or members of the media may ask you questions about the disaster or the response. Refer all such requests to the designated spokesperson for your facility. If you are assigned to answer questions and provide information (for example, through a hotline), you will receive training and written materials to guide you.

Imagine that a chemical agent has had widespread release and that thousands of people need to be decontaminated. State and local emergency management agencies will work with health departments to provide ongoing public education. They might describe what citizens could do and expect to have happen during decontamination, such as removing clothing and taking showers. Often, they will read a prepared statement.

Incidents that involve environmental threats or terrorism are particularly troubling to the public. No one knows for sure about the long-term health consequences. When people do not get answers or do not get the answers that they want, they can become angry. Effective communication that involves empathetic listening can help build trust and calm people.

Communicating with Patients about Their Personal Risks

Healthcare personnel can be helpful in reducing anxiety, confusion, and panic among patients who have experienced trauma or exposure to chemicals or infectious disease. Your communication skills as a health professional are important during and after an emergency or disaster. Healthcare professionals may be asked about:

- Current information concerning the cause of the incident or status of help

- Potential short- and long-term effects of the disaster
- Potential short- and long-term effects of the patient condition
- Recommended patient treatment
- Other relevant information, such as ongoing risk

Before you provide any information, check the facts. Be sure that your source is reliable and that everything that you communicate corresponds with what the public officials and spokespersons are communicating. Also, stay within the scope of your practice. You should not be communicating anything about a patient's conditions or treatments beyond what has already been told to them by their providers. You would only need to affirm and repeat their counsel.

If there is panic or anger, demonstrate assurance and calmness. By keeping cool, health professionals can help patients and others stay calm and work together to solve problems.

A Closer Look

Steps in Risk Communication

1. Be empathetic. Show concern for patients and their families.
2. Listen to patients. Try to understand their concerns. Even if patients do not have a perfect understanding of what has happened, you want to understand how the events are affecting their lives.
3. Tell patients that they were right to seek medical care.
4. Provide as much information as possible in a way that the patients will understand.
5. Help patients comply with treatment.

Point of Dispensing Sites

In public health emergencies involving infectious diseases, there may be a need for mass distributions of immunizations, antidotes, or medications. This is called **mass prophylaxis** and is conducted to reduce the spread of disease.

There are two approaches to distribution: "push" and "pull." The push approach involves having health workers bring medicine to the patients. The pull approach is to have the patients come to the health workers. The most efficient way is to invite them to a central location.

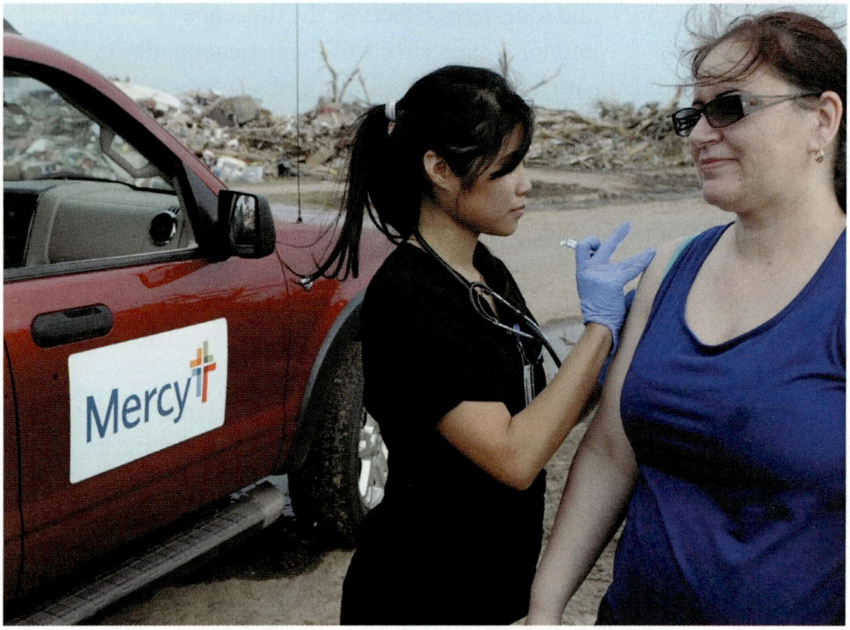

A nurse from Mercy Hospital provides a resident in Moore, Oklahoma, with a tetanus shot as a prophylactic treatment after a tornado ripped through the neighborhood.

If local authorities along with the state department of health and the CDC decide there is a need for mass prophylaxis, a **Point of Dispensing** (POD) site may be set up. A POD is a temporary station for dispensing vaccines and preventive medications, or antidotes for chemical exposures. Patients do not pay for the medications dispensed through a POD—they are paid for by public health funds. The POD may be supported by the city, county, or state DOH, or the CDC if a presidential disaster declaration has been made.

HHS may also declare a public health emergency requiring a POD if a disease, disorder, or bioterrorist attack is threatening the public's health. A declaration of a public health emergency allows HHS to use its operational funds to set up PODs in areas where they are needed without a presidential declaration. The CDC works with the state, county, and/or city health departments to set up the PODs.

Point of Dispensing Setup and Staffing

An attempt is made to establish the POD sites in "easy-to-reach" locations large enough to accommodate the expected number of patients. A POD should be set up to promote a controlled flow of people and efficient service. There should be a logical path through the POD site, with entrances and exits clearly marked.

A POD site requires both medical personnel and large numbers of support workers. Since workers must be mobilized quickly, it is important that volunteers preregister with their local health department to be part of a POD team. Allied health professionals are likely to fill many roles as employees and volunteers. Emergency Medical Service personnel (EMTs and paramedics) or DMATs (if activated) may need to do triage at the POD to separate those who have not been exposed to the infectious disease from those who have. They may also be involved in screening people who might be allergic to the medication or vaccination being dispensed, or have a contraindication or a symptom or condition that makes it inadvisable to receive it.

Be Aware

A Point of Distribution (POD) site, which provides citizens access to emergency supplies, is not the same as a Point of Dispensing (POD) site, even though they share the same acronym. Be careful not to confuse them.

A Closer Look

Roles for Health Professionals at Point of Dispensing Sites

Some of the roles for health professionals at a POD site are:

- **Greeters:** Direct people into the POD, provide basic information, and screen for visibly ill people who require immediate medical evaluation
- **Forms Distributors:** Hand out and collect patient forms used in triage and follow-up, hand out patient information sheets on medications or immunizations
- **Triage Supporters:** Identify people requiring medical or behavioral health evaluation, identify drug allergies and contraindications for treatments
- **Immunizers:** Administer medication
- **Immunizer Assistants:** Check supplies, prepare injection site, apply dressing, provide patients with instructions
- **Emergency Medical Service personnel:** Evaluate and stabilize any ill patients, if present; respond to medical emergencies, if needed
- **Transportation Assistants:** Move patients to ambulances, buses, or vans to be transported to a medical facility
- **Medication Dispensers:** Repackage medications, determine correct medication types and doses for both adults and children
- **Recovery Area Staff:** Help people who have reactions to the medication or vaccine
- **Forms Collection and Exit:** Check patient contact information, advise on follow-up care, check that patients received the correct medication

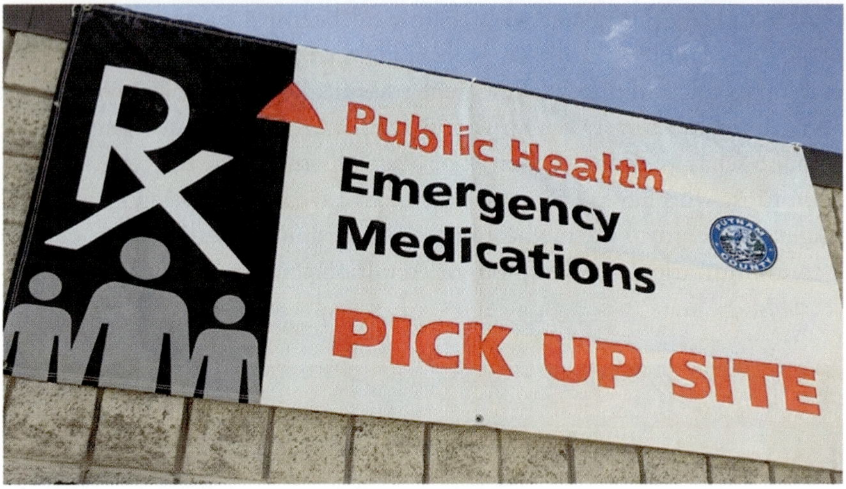

In New York State, the Putnam County Department of Health held a POD drill in Brewster, having 350 county employees role-play that they were patients needing life-saving medications. The county DOH collaborated with the county Bureau of Emergency Services and the Sheriff's Department for this August 18, 2015, event.

Some counties also run mobile Point of Dispensing units, which are a mix of both the push and the pull approach, as they ask residents to come to a central neighborhood location where the unit will be parked.

Strategic National Stockpile

The medications or immunizations disbursed through a POD are likely to come from the federal government through a program called the **Strategic National Stockpile (SNS)**. The SNS is a federally run massive storage system, or bank, of medicines, vaccines, antidotes, and related medical supplies. The SNS provides the vaccines and antidotes for POD sites, but it also sends out the preventive medical supplies and medications for the federal medical teams and hospitals in natural disasters.

Maintained by the CDC, the SNS has large quantities of **push packs**. Push packs are ready-to-deploy containers with enough medical supplies and medications to treat thousands of patients. There are different types of packs based on the type of need, disease, or disaster situation, such as fighting bacterial and viral diseases, pandemic influenza, radiation/nuclear emergencies, or chemical attacks. These medications for prevention or antidotes are known as **medical countermeasures**.

HHS conducts an annual review of the stockpile's formulary and determines which types of push packs and items to include based on US public health tracking data and current disease threats. The local authorities work with the DOH and the CDC to determine the types of push packs needed for the community.

There are also push packs for general medical needs and for treating trauma from disasters. Push packs can be delivered to any state within 12 hours.

The large containers of drugs, vaccines, medical supplies, and equipment are delivered by air or by ground transportation in two phases. In the first phase of a response to a natural disaster, the CDC staff managing the SNS will send the affected area push packages that contain 50 tons of a broad range of pharmaceuticals and medical supplies that are prepacked. Each state has emergency plans for receiving and distributing the medicine and supplies to local communities.

When an SNS push pack arrives, the state sends teams, including pharmacists and pharmacy technicians, to the arrival site to inventory and accept the shipment. The team repackages the inventory into smaller packs that are distributed to medical teams or healthcare sites, or the pharmaceutical PODs. If needed, the stockpile can also send a Federal Medical Station Strike Team along with the inventory. This team is a group of specialists that can help assist in setting up the POD and providing on-the-spot training for POD volunteers.

In addition, the SNS can provide a temporary Federal Medical Station (FMS). These medical stations operate as short-term hospitals. The Federal Medical Station is equipped with enough beds, supplies, medicines, and equipment for three days before it needs to be restocked. The Federal Medical Station will be staffed by members of a DMAT.

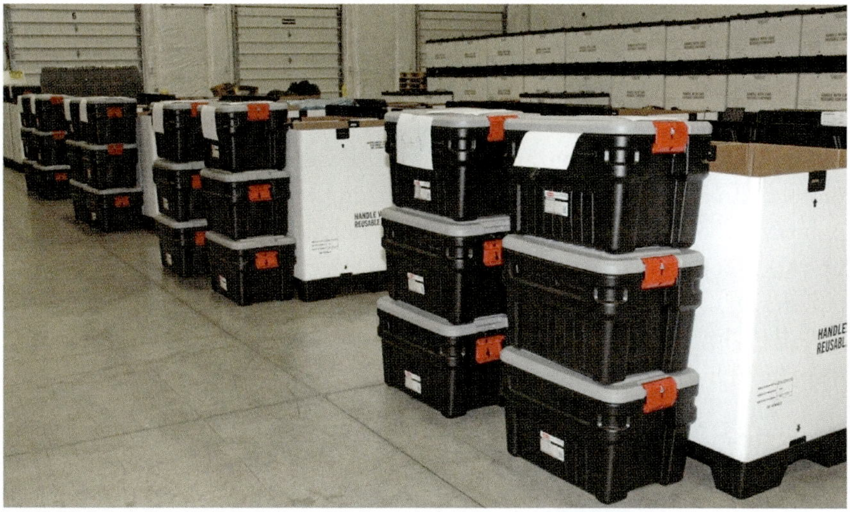

Local, county, state, and tribal authorities can request assistance from the SNS for public health emergencies or threats. In 2015, the SNS assembled containers that contained PPE kits to be worn by emergency responders when administering treatments to patients with Ebola Virus Disease. Each kit contained enough PPE supplies to protect a healthcare professional caring for a patient with Ebola Virus Disease for up to five days.

If it appears that these additional resources will not be enough to meet the medical need, the CDC could implement the second phase, which might require an Emergency Use Authorization. Additional medications and supplies are sent by the manufacturers under contract with the federal government.

Handling Healthcare Facility Waste

Be Aware

When dealing with highly infectious diseases—such as EVD—bedding and personal protective equipment is considered medical waste.

During usual operations at any hospital, a large amount of waste is generated. However, during an epidemic, CBRNE incident, or natural disaster with many patients needing medical care, there will be even more healthcarewaste that must be handled properly. The failure to do so, even at temporary medical stations, could hinder the ability to control the spread of toxic exposure or infection.

Healthcare waste includes general medications and hazardous chemicals used in medical procedures or treatments, such as chemotherapy and nuclear medications, radiological dyes for diagnosis, and biohazardous compounds, such as bioengineered drugs, hormone agents, and antiviral drugs. It also includes infectious waste, which encompasses any materials that may carry or have been exposed to infectious substances. In a healthcare facility, the term **medical waste** (or *regulated medical waste*) is used to describe its infectious or potentially infectious waste, such as body fluids or blood products; laboratory specimens from various procedures or biopsies; bandages and diapers; and the PPE used when caring for patients with highly infectious diseases. The clothes of patients who have been exposed to biological toxins must also be considered hazardous and be discarded following the hospital's protocol. In addition, used **sharps**, or anything with a sharp, cutting edge or point, must be collected as dangerous and potentially infectious and picked up for disposal. Sharps include hypodermic needles, syringes, scalpels, and pipettes.

All healthcare waste must be handled and disposed of carefully to prevent a potential hazard to public health.

Treating Healthcare Waste

There are two primary methods for treating nonsharps infectious waste so that it is no longer hazardous: incineration and autoclaving. **Incineration** is the burning of waste at temperatures ranging from 1,800° F to 2,000° F (982° C to 1,093° C). **Autoclaving** (also known as steam sterilization) exposes the waste to steam at sufficient temperature and pressure and for a long enough time to ensure that microorganisms are destroyed. Nonsharps infectious waste is treated on-site or by outside contractors.

During an emergency or disaster, a key priority is the collection and treatment of infectious waste, because it may become more infectious over time. All infectious waste must be treated within seven days. Many facilities have autoclaves for sterilizing their own medical waste. However, when power is lost, the hospital may not be able to allocate a generator for medical waste. As a result, waste can accumulate before it can be treated or removed. If it is not possible to keep up with the treatment of medical waste, and power and freezer space are available, healthcare facilities may consider freezing medical waste temporarily.

In addition to handling their own waste, hospital incinerators sometimes treat the medical waste of private medical practices. In an emergency or disaster, if the hospital incinerator is working, it can provide a valuable service to the community by incinerating the medical waste of other medical providers. They may not be able to keep up with all the increased volume and may need outside assistance.

Sharps waste should be collected when containers are three-fourths full. If transportation is not available, new containers can be designated while waiting for pick up to resume.

Chemical and nuclear wastes are generally handled and disposed of separately from other healthcare waste—hazardous or nuclear waste companies usually handle the disposal.

Transportation issues can affect the treatment of healthcare waste. If transportation is disrupted, different kinds of waste can build up to dangerous levels. In its emergency and disaster plan, each facility includes alternative procedures for collecting, sorting, transporting, and disposing of waste.

Procedures for Reopening a Hospital or Clinic

After an emergency or disaster, in addition to handling waste, a hospital or medical facility has to meet a number of requirements before it can reopen the facility or any portion that was damaged. Before doing any repair, personnel must survey the facility to carefully document the losses and damage for possible reimbursement from insurance or FEMA. Once repairs are completed, a medical physicist needs to evaluate any equipment that required major repair, was disassembled and reassembled, or was replaced to ensure that equipment is working properly. The local and state health inspectors must inspect the facility. The Joint Commission would also need to be notified about any healthcare facility that was forced to close due to a disaster. The accrediting body will then decide what is needed to ensure that the facility meets accreditation standards before it reopens.

Departments and clinics need to do the same thing. For example, under the Mammography Quality Standards Act, personnel of an imaging facility that performs mammograms would have to inform its accrediting organization and the state health department as soon as possible that it is ready to reopen and possibly have the department reaccredited.

When facilities and departments reopen after damage or shutdowns, communication to the public and patients is key. It restores trust and a return to normal functioning. When the healthcare facilities and their services are known to be fully restored, the whole community feels one step further down the path to recovery.

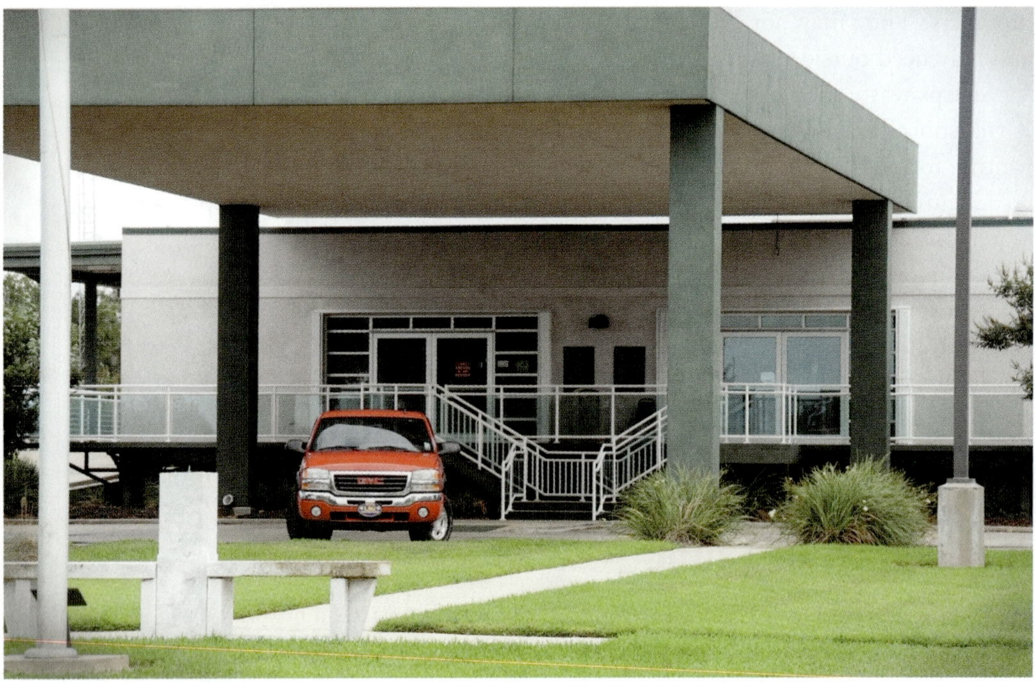

This 2013 view of the South Cameron Memorial Hospital in Louisiana shows a hospital transformation. The hospital was severely damaged in 2005 during Hurricane Rita. Through the help of FEMA's Public Assistance Grant Program, the hospital was replaced with a new structure that is raised ten feet above the flood level to protect against future damage.

Chapter Summary

Health professionals have many important roles in the tasks involved in emergency and disaster response. They support triage procedures that are used to quickly evaluate a large number of victims. They follow the standard protocols and universal precautions to prevent the spread of disease. Controlling the spread of contamination is always critical, especially during an emergency or disaster. Healthcare facilities have procedures that must be followed to control and treat contamination, and to isolate or quarantine people.

When communicating to the public about the risks of an emergency, disaster, or infectious disease, great care must be taken. Public spokespeople deliver information intended to help the public take the proper actions. Allied health professionals can assist in communicating effectively by knowing what the spokespeople have said and providing accurate information to patients in a calm manner. Allied health professionals may also work at a Point of Dispensing site, where many people receive immunizations, medicines, or antidotes in response to a public health emergency.

To prevent spreading the toxic or infectious substances, hospitals must properly handle and treat its different types of waste. Once repairs have been made to a healthcare facility, then it must go through inspections and reaccreditation to reopen. When the time is right, the spokespeople must communicate to the public that the risk is over and it is time to return for excellent care.

Key Terms	
antidote	mass prophylaxis
ambulatory	medical countermeasures
autoclaving	medical waste
cohorted patients	Point of Dispensing
contaminated patient	push pack
cold zone	quarantine
decontamination	respirator
don and doff	risk communication
droplet precautions	sharps
fit tested	social distancing
hot zone	triage
incineration	universal precautions
infection control procedures	warm zone
isolation	

Additional Resources

To extend the content presented in this chapter, take advantage of the resources available through the chapter's eBook resource links and the end-of-chapter link. These resources include informational supplements and flash cards for terms and abbreviations.

Recognizing Terms

Choose the word or phrase from the list of key terms that best matches each of the following descriptions. Your instructor may ask you to submit your work for grading or may provide you with an answer key for self-assessment.

1. The area with the most exposure to a hazardous agent, where it is most dangerous to be __________
2. Hand washing, wearing protective clothing and gear, using good hygiene __________
3. Container of drugs, vaccines, medical supplies __________
4. Communicating information about a health crisis in a timely, accurate manner __________
5. Substance that can counteract a form of disease or poison __________
6. Used hypodermic needles, syringes, scalpels, pipettes __________
7. Procedure that exposes medical waste to steam at sufficient temperature and pressure and for a long enough time to ensure that microorganisms are destroyed __________
8. Mask designed to prevent the inhalation of very small particles, such as viruses, harmful dust, fumes, vapors, or gases __________
9. Patients with similar symptoms who are grouped together in a hospital __________
10. Temporary station for dispensing antidotes for chemical exposure, vaccines, and medications __________

Reviewing Concepts

Choose the response that best answers the question or completes the sentence. Your instructor may ask you to submit your work for grading or may provide you with an answer key for self-assessment.

1. How many patients could a two-person triage team be able to assess in 10 minutes?
   a. five
   b. twenty
   c. fifty
   d. two
2. What does the START system use to categorize level of care?
   a. number code
   b. temperature code
   c. color code
   d. alphanumeric code
3. During an emergency or disaster, litter bearers
   a. conduct triage.
   b. pick up hazardous debris.
   c. transport victims on stretchers.
   d. drive ambulances to hospitals.
4. Victims of a disaster can go to a Point of Dispensing site to receive
   a. information on the location of family members.
   b. a vaccination.
   c. FEMA-disbursed cash.
   d. a voucher for housing assistance.
5. What is one role of an emergency medical technician at a Point of Dispensing site?
   a. direct people into the POD
   b. hand out forms used in triage
   c. evaluate ill patients
   d. repackage medications
6. Which organization establishes standard and universal precautions?
   a. Centers for Disease Control and Prevention
   b. American Red Cross
   c. Occupational Safety and Health Administration
   d. National Institutes of Health

7. Which item of personal protective equipment requires fit testing?
   a. moon suit
   b. N95 respirator mask
   c. nonlatex glove
   d. medical mask

8. A patient with tuberculosis should be
   a. isolated.
   b. liberated.
   c. decontaminated.
   d. cohorted.

9. To which laboratory in the Laboratory Response Network should a suspected bioterrorist agent be sent?
   a. sentinel laboratory
   b. reference laboratory
   c. national laboratory
   d. international laboratory

10. A method of cleaning medical waste using steam is
    a. autoclaving.
    b. incineration.
    c. mass prophylaxis.
    d. decontamination.

11. During an emergency, which type of waste should receive first priority in collection and treatment?
    a. sharps waste
    b. biohazardous waste
    c. documents containing private information
    d. food waste

12. What is the minimum temperature required for incineration of medical waste?
    a. 212° F
    b. 800° F
    c. 1,800° F
    d. 18,000° F

13. Why is it important to use social distancing techniques?
    a. Social distancing is an effective way to communicate.
    b. Federal law requires the use of social distancing techniques.
    c. Social distancing helps people get along better.
    d. Social distancing techniques reduce the transmission of an infectious disease.

14. When an SNS push pack arrives, what happens? (Select all that apply.)
    a. The state sends teams to inventory and accept the shipment.
    b. The team repackages the inventory into smaller packs.
    c. The packs are distributed to medical teams, healthcare sites, or PODs.
    d. Healthcare professionals have people come to their private doctors to receive the medication.

15. What is the warm zone in decontamination? (Select all that apply.)
    a. An area next to the hot zone where patients can cool off.
    b. An area, at least 300 feet and upwind and uphill from the incident, designated for the decontamination of patients.
    c. An area where patients are sorted into treatment categories.
    d. An area where ambulatory patients walk to change their clothes.

Exploring Emergency Preparedness Issues

Complete the following activities to further explore the concepts found in this chapter. Your instructor may ask you to submit your work for grading or may provide you with guidance for self-assessment.

1. Contact a local hospital. Find out about its procedures to isolate or quarantine patients. Will these procedures change in the event of pandemic influenza? Does its plan for an episode of pandemic influenza have a specific task that will be performed by your health profession? Discuss what you learn in a one- to two-page report.

2. Contact a medical laboratory in your community. Is it part of the Laboratory Response Network? Has it handled a "suspicious sample?" What were the tasks carried out by your health profession? Where is the reference laboratory in your region? Summarize this information in a one-page report.

3. Contact the local EMS agency in your community. Find out about its procedures for decontaminating victims in the field. How often has it had to use these procedures in the past two years? What equipment is used to communicate with the local hospital? Does your hospital include your health profession in its plan to decontaminate patients? If yes, what are the tasks? Summarize what you learn in a two-page report.

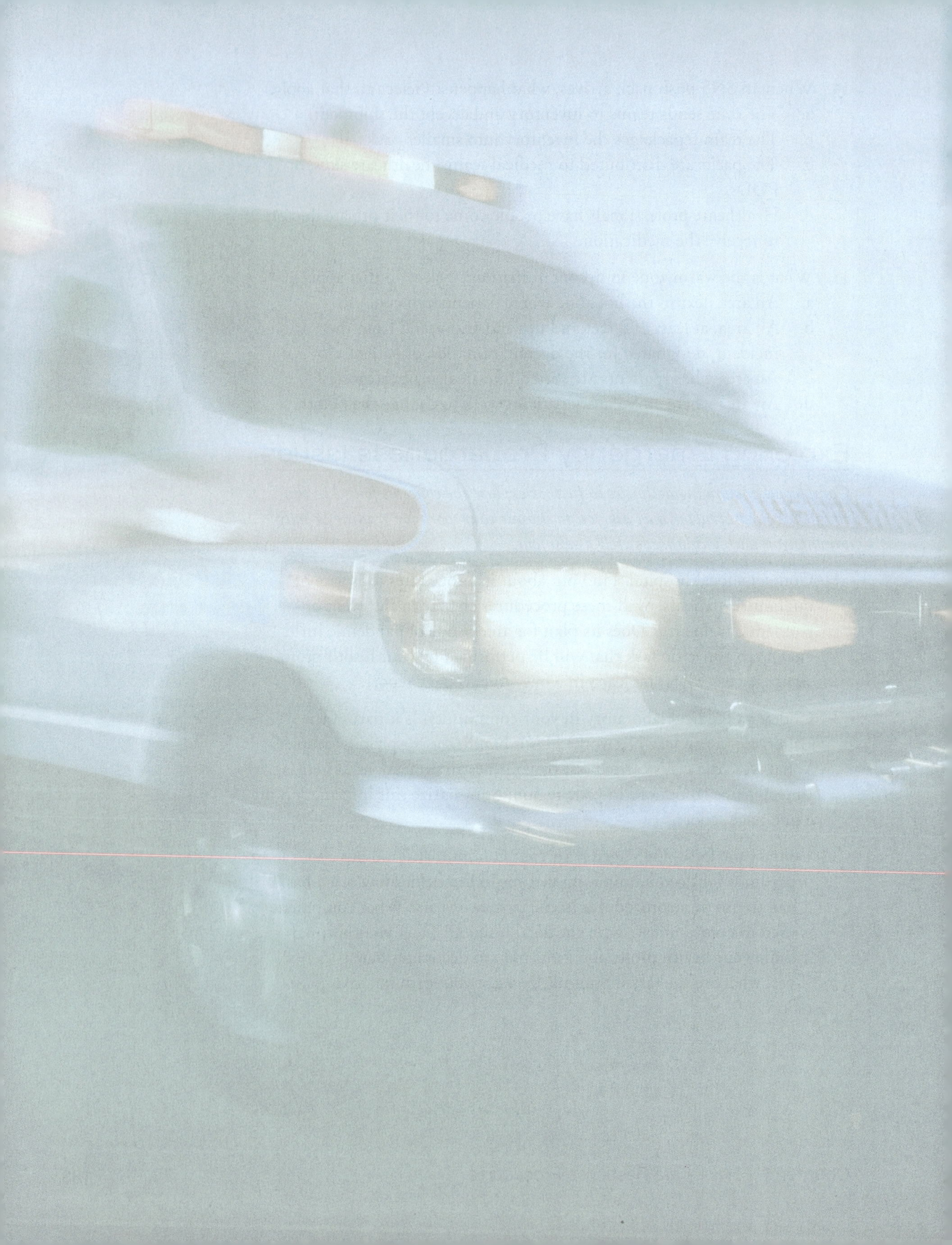

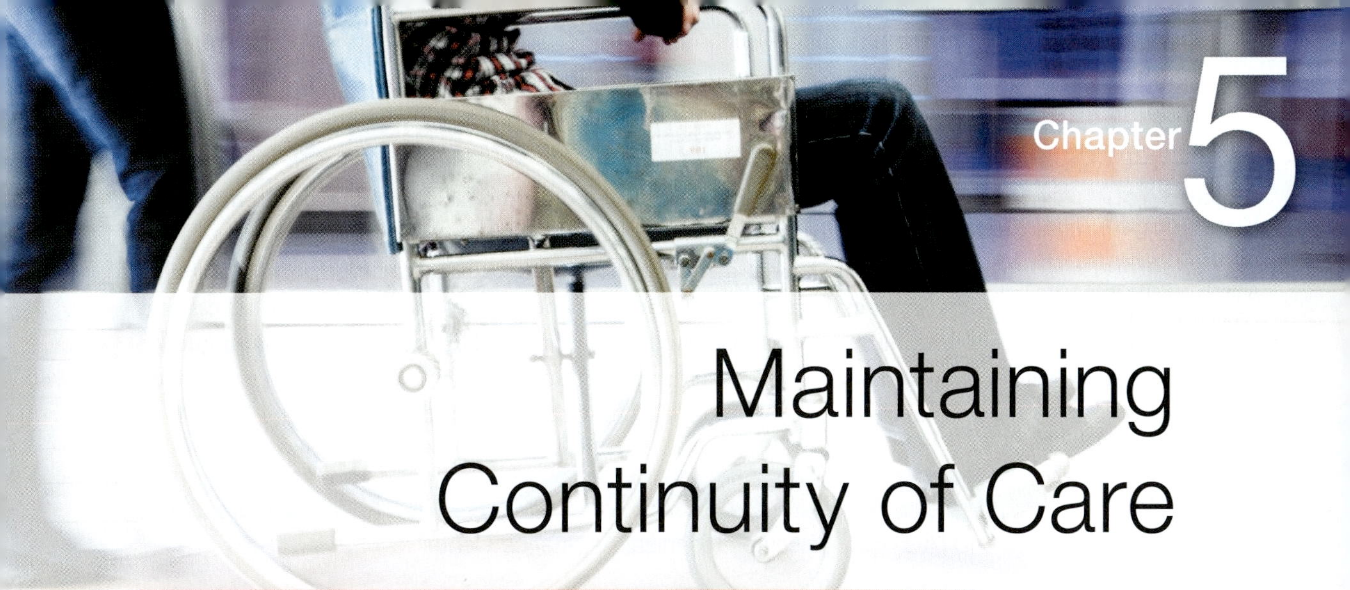

Chapter 5

Maintaining Continuity of Care

What You Will Learn

- Why continuity of care is important during and after an emergency or disaster
- Considerations for at-risk populations during and after an emergency or disaster
- How to advise patients with chronic diseases to prepare for and cope with disasters
- What medical shelters are, how they are staffed, and how they operate
- How behavioral health services are provided
- Resources for animals and pets in an emergency or disaster

When we think about health-related problems and disasters, we usually think about injuries and illnesses that are the direct result of a disaster. We rarely think about how disasters affect at-risk populations, patients with chronic diseases, and health issues on a broader scale. For example, people who are chronically ill have special health needs that may not be met or met easily during and after a disaster. Without access to the healthcare system for continuity of care, individuals with these conditions are likely to get sicker. **Continuity of care** is ongoing, coordinated medical care received from the same group of healthcare professionals. Continuity of care is often interrupted following a disaster. The reestablishment of healthcare systems should be a priority for communities so that normal care can resume.

Caring for At-Risk Individuals

> **Expand Your Knowledge**
>
> Working together, the American Red Cross and FEMA created the guide "Preparing for Disaster for People with Disabilities and Other Special Needs." You can access it at: **EmDPrp2.ParadigmEducation.com/SpecialNeedsPrep**.
>
> FEMA also has preparation tips and online tools for individuals with access and functional needs: **EmDPrp2.ParadigmEducation.com/access-functional-needs**.

The elderly, people with disabilities, children, and people who do not speak English have unique healthcare needs during and after a disaster. These groups are considered **at-risk populations** because they are particularly vulnerable to experiencing difficulties. These individuals may have access and functional needs, as discussed in Chapter 3. Health professionals should be aware of the challenges that at-risk populations experience during emergency and disaster response and know how to help them.

Key Acronyms	
DTAC	Disaster Technical Assistance Center
EIF	emergency information form
EPAP	Emergency Prescription Assistance Program
NACA	National Animal Care & Control Association
NDARRT	National Disaster Animal Response and Recovery Team
SAMHSA	Substance Abuse and Mental Health Services Administration
VMAT	Veterinary Medical Assistance Team

Elderly and People with Disabilities

Elderly patients, especially those who live on their own, are particularly at risk in disasters. If they are not paying attention to media, they may not be aware of any danger. When roads or subways are damaged, nursing aides and/or family members may not be able to help them. Besides medical care, elderly patients may require help with meals or transportation. Many seniors function well and don't require services to live independently. However, without power, they are at risk. Older adults also tend to be more sensitive to extremes of hot and cold weather as when heat or air conditioning is disrupted.

Adults of other ages who have limited mobility or who are hearing or visually impaired may need help finding medical care. They may have difficulty learning about the incident or what to do. For example, after Hurricane Katrina, many people who were hearing impaired did not know about orders to evacuate. Because the power was out, they could not follow closed-captioned television announcements. Cell phone text messaging also did not work.

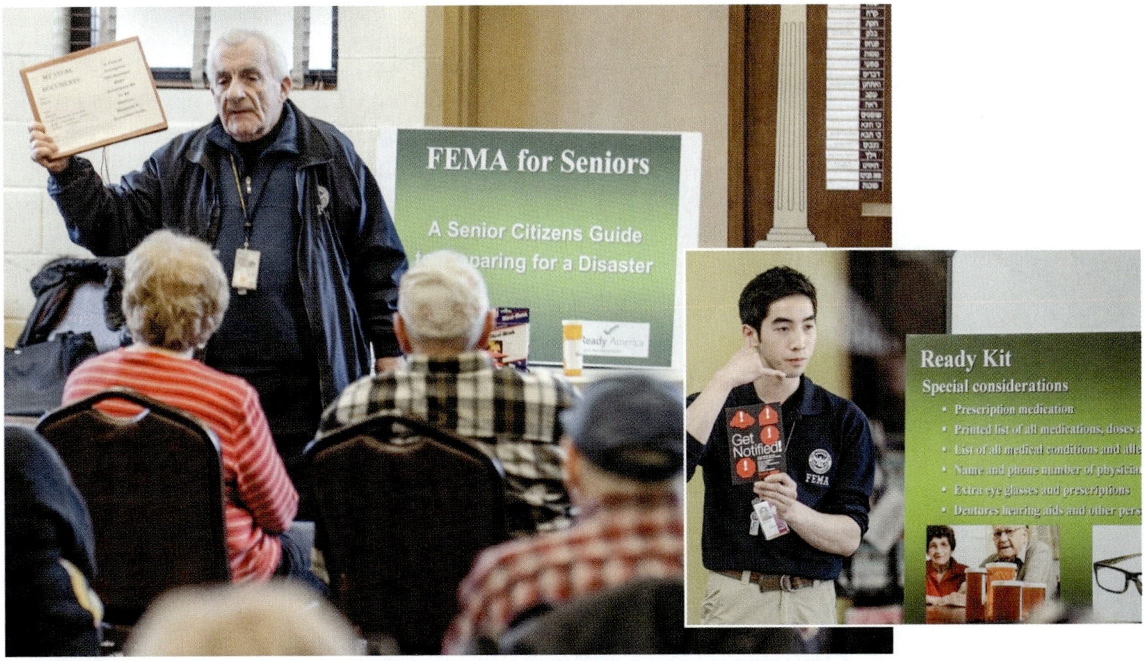

In April 2013, FEMA offered presentations on emergency preparedness at a senior center in New York. The presentations encouraged participants to make an emergency kit and a list of their medications and other emergency information.

A Closer Look

Seniors in Hurricane Sandy

During Hurricane Sandy, 17% of New York City's population was age 60 years or older. Senior citizens living in Manhattan were stuck in high-rise buildings when the elevators did not work because of power failure. Some of these seniors required food and water. Volunteers and health department personnel carried these necessities up many flights of stairs to reach them.

More than 70% (31 of the 44 deaths) of those who died during Hurricane Sandy were seniors, or 55 years or older. Most drowned at home because they did not evacuate. Their failure to evacuate was due in part to not knowing that they needed to leave or why. Neighbors evacuated without informing them or checking on them.

Some seniors felt safer in their homes. Some stayed in their apartments so that they could help others who had not evacuated, such as cooking for the families with young children in their building and checking on other seniors to be sure that they were safe. Other seniors took leadership roles in training volunteers or helped identify isolated seniors who might need extra help.

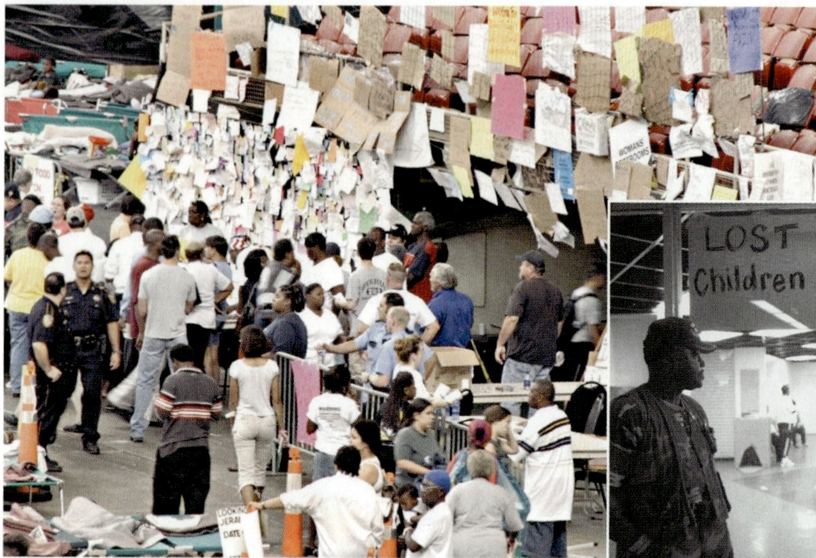

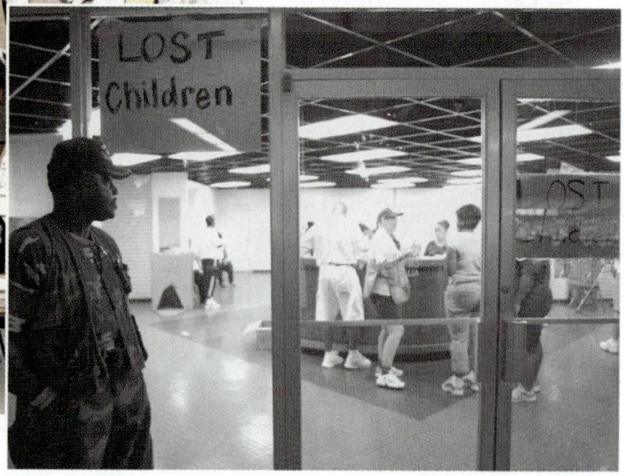

Approximately 18,000 Hurricane Katrina evacuees were housed at Houston's Astrodome and Reliant Center after evacuating New Orleans. Many were still looking for their loved ones. They checked the lost children center and the message board set up by the American Red Cross in the Reliant Center.

Children

Children are at risk in a disaster because, to them, the situation is confusing and frightening. They often have difficulty adjusting when living temporarily in an evacuation center or other temporary housing without their daily routine, including school. In addition, children need the support of friends and relatives who may not be with them. If injured, they may require medical equipment that has been designed specifically for children, and medications that are adjusted for their body size. These medical modifications and devices can be harder to locate (or may not be available) in disaster situations. In addition, children typically cannot receive medical treatment without parental permission. Facilities usually have protocols for treating children whose parents are not present.

Children with chronic medical conditions are in greater danger when a disaster disables healthcare systems. They need to be able to see their regular doctors and receive treatments on time to prevent their conditions from getting worse. Many pediatricians who care for children with chronic conditions prepare an **emergency information form (EIF)**, which summarizes the medical conditions, medications, and other needed information about these children.

Typically, children spend much of their day away from their parents, in school. Families may be separated when a disaster hits. If separated, children will be unable to care for themselves. For instance, in Hurricane Katrina, there were more than 5,000 cases of missing children. Some were separated for weeks, and some for months.

As part of their all-hazards emergency preparedness plans, communities need to develop procedures for the **reunification**, or bringing back together, of children and their families. This may include evacuation tracking systems and ways for parents and children to contact each other as part of the evacuation shelters. The American Red Cross helps reunite children and families.

Pediatricians can talk to parents and guardians about making emergency and reunification plans. Health professionals should get to know their facility's emergency procedures for reuniting children with their families and guardians. Many organizations and individuals use social media tools to assist in this reunification. (More information on personal, family, and neighborhood preparation is presented in Chapter 6.)

Expand Your Knowledge

The American Red Cross has the Safe and Well program, where victims can register and let people know they are safe. It can be viewed at: **http:// EmDPrp2. ParadigmEducation.com/ SaveandWellProgram**.

For more uses of social media for emergency and disaster communications, see the eBook supplement "Social Media Tools Used in Emergency and Disaster Communications."

Immigrants and Non-English Speakers

People who speak limited or no English are another at-risk group, especially if they are injured or separated from loved ones and have no one to translate for them. Federal regulations require hospitals and other healthcare facilities to provide interpreters (translators) in the many different languages used locally and in American sign language. Healthcare organizations and nonprofits that serve a significant number of people for whom English is not their primary language can help their patients by providing preprepared and translated information on emergencies. In these communities, elders often have not yet mastered the language.

Expand Your Knowledge

You can learn more about communicating with non-English-speaking and multicultural patients in the eBook supplement entitled "Tips for Working in a Multicultural Healthcare Environment."

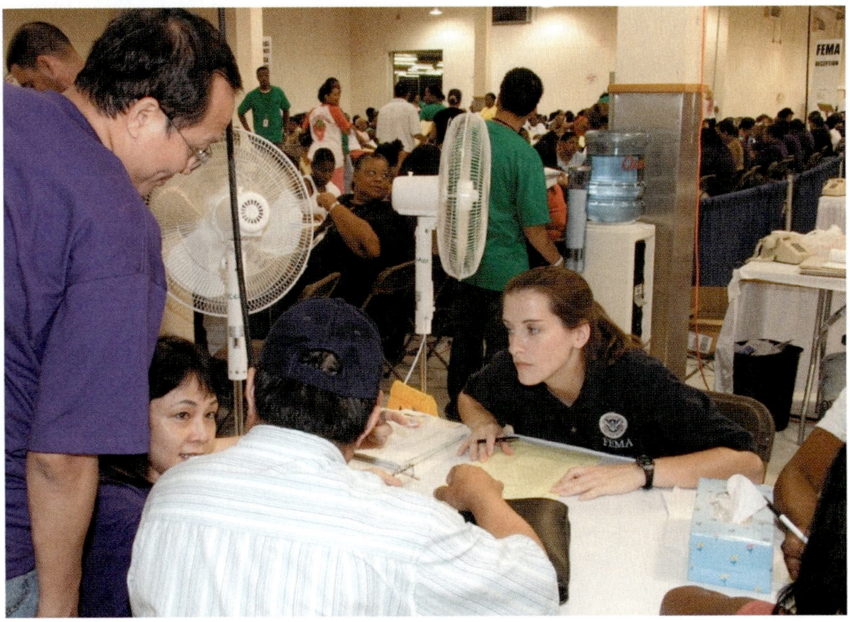

In Houston at the Disaster Recovery Center (DRC), Vietnamese interpreters assist a FEMA representative in providing disaster relief services to Hurricane Katrina victims on September 28, 2005. The DRC provided interpreters for several languages, including American Sign Language.

Patients with Chronic Conditions

As explained in earlier chapters, disasters may disrupt the delivery of health-care services, and chronically ill patients are at risk if they have not prepared ahead of time. Certain health complications can be expected and planned for. For example, patients with cardiovascular conditions may have higher blood pressure or unstable angina during or immediately after an emergency or disaster, thereby increasing the risk of myocardial infarction (heart attack) or stroke. People with asthma and other pulmonary conditions may have problems triggered by exposure to mold, smoke, or airborne pathogens. People with diabetes are particularly vulnerable to infection if they get an open cut or wound. Other patients with certain medical conditions, such as lupus, or medication treatments, such as chemotherapy, can also have lower immunity and be more susceptible to an infectious disease.

A Closer Look

Diabetes during Hurricane Katrina

Whether in a disaster or not, individuals with diabetes must be able to monitor their glucose levels and diets, have supplies of insulin, and get physical activity. They must be very careful to prevent development or worsening of hypertension, dyslipidemia, and other related conditions. Imagine how difficult this is in an evacuation shelter—especially if patients do not have sufficient supplies or insulin and do not have medical or medication records with them. In addition, diabetic patients are more susceptible to infection, and in floods, many evacuees, who may have skin abrasions, might wade through contaminated water. This can lead to serious infections.

At the time of Hurricane Katrina, more than 10% of the population in some affected areas of New Orleans was diabetic. Evacuees with diabetes may have been able to take their insulin with them but they often lacked supplies or a way to keep their insulin properly refrigerated in the intense heat. Other patients may have accessed insulin dispensed by a Disaster Medical Assistance Team (DMAT), but the insulin may not have matched what they were usually prescribed. Some patients only had the insulin supplies that they had brought with them when they evacuated.

To provide supplies for diabetic patients living in shelters, the Pennington Biomedical Research Center started a collection program, called Diabetes Relief, to gather glucose monitors, lancets, glucose tablets/gel, alcohol preps, and insulin pumps. Pharmacies that could remain open tried to fill the needed prescriptions on an emergency basis.

Providing Prescribed Medications and Medical Supplies

Accessing medications during an emergency or disaster is clearly an ongoing need for chronically ill populations because many patients are not prepared for the disruption in healthcare services. For instance, following Hurricane Sandy, thousands of people were displaced from their homes without their needed prescriptions. Some went to hospital emergency departments to get medications. Others received prescriptions for conditions diagnosed by a medical provider at a DMAT. Even if they found an open pharmacy, many individuals could not access their money because of banking problems or because their paychecks were not deposited as usual due to businesses being shut down. Some patients could not pay the copay for their pharmacy prescriptions. To address these issues during the disaster period, several national pharmacy chains waived the copays.

For the uninsured, pharmacies that are enrolled in the federal government's **Emergency Prescription Assistance Program (EPAP)** can provide a 30-day supply of prescribed medications, specific medical supplies, vaccines, and certain medical equipment during a federally designated disaster. This coverage can be renewed every 30 days, as long as the EPAP is active.

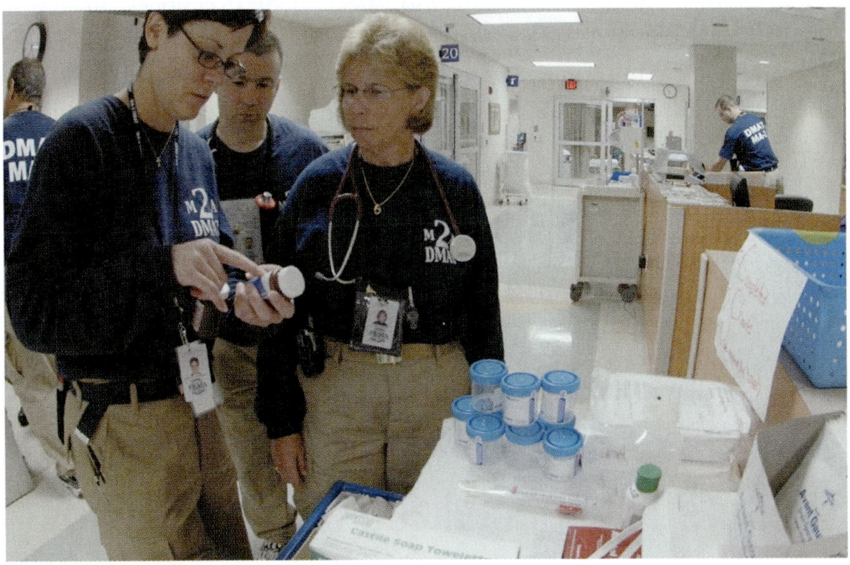

In response to Hurricane Dennis in July 2005, the Massachusetts-2-DMAT staff members check a patient's medication. The DMAT came to Sacred Heart Hospital in Pensacola, Florida, to assist with the medical surge of patients needing care.

Expand Your Knowledge

Currently, more than 70,000 pharmacies participate in the EPAP. For more information on the EPAP, go to http://EmDPrp2.ParadigmEducation.com/EPAP.

Replacing lost medications can also be a problem during and after a disaster. Prescription insurance plans often limit the number of refills or the amount of medication that can be dispensed in a single month. If a person has already had a prescription filled, the insurance company may not pay for a refill that month. These issues need to be worked out with the individual insurance companies. Patients eligible for the EPAP can initiate a claim for certain medical items if they were lost, stolen, or destroyed as the result of qualifying disasters.

Even if patients have their prescribed medications, there can still be issues. As noted earlier, some medications must be protected from heat and direct sunlight, and most patients are aware of this. If the electrical power has been off for a long time, medications that require refrigeration may have to be discarded. Other medications that require refrigeration may still be viable, but they will have a shorter **shelf life**, which is the amount of time a medication is usable before it reaches its expiration date.

Package inserts for medications and supplies often provide information about what to do if the medication has not been properly refrigerated. For this reason, patients should be encouraged to keep package inserts or the original medication containers (though the pharmacies or manufacturers can provide package inserts, the information can also be found online).

Healthcare professionals should inform and remind patients that extremes of temperature and humidity can also affect medical supplies, including blood glucose monitors and test strips. For example, diagnostic tests, including blood glucose tests, may not be accurate if the meter is damaged. Meters should be discarded if they have been exposed to unusually high temperatures for more than 24 hours.

Any medications that have, or may have, come in contact with contaminated water should be discarded. Medical supplies also need to be uncontaminated, such as blood glucose meters and test strips, sterile gauze and wound dressings, disposable thermometers, syringes, and tubing. They should be used only if the packaging is dry and intact and the contents are still sterile and untouched by moisture. Patients should consult with a pharmacist or supplier of durable medical devices about whether to dispose of a device if it has been touched by floodwaters.

Shelters for Specialized Medical Needs

There are many patients with more complex or serious medical conditions who cannot be properly cared for in the evacuation shelters set up for the general population. A **medical shelter** is an evacuation shelter outfitted with some medical staff and equipment. State health departments are responsible for setting up these specialized temporary facilities after any disaster involving evacuations. This kind of shelter serves people who:

- Have acute medical conditions that require professional evaluation, assessment, and maintenance
- Require skilled nursing care but not hospitalization (though not all states allow these patients into their medical shelters because they do not have enough staff)

The setup, mission, and operation of medical shelters range widely from state to state. To serve their patients, these specialized shelters need a refrigerator and cabinets for the storage of medication, and they must be equipped to properly store and use oxygen.

Expand Your Knowledge

In 2017, HHS deployed medical assets in advance of Hurricane Harvey. This preparation included the use of 500 Federal Medical Station (FMS) beds, 6 DMATs, 460 NDMS staff, and 1 Coordinated Response team.

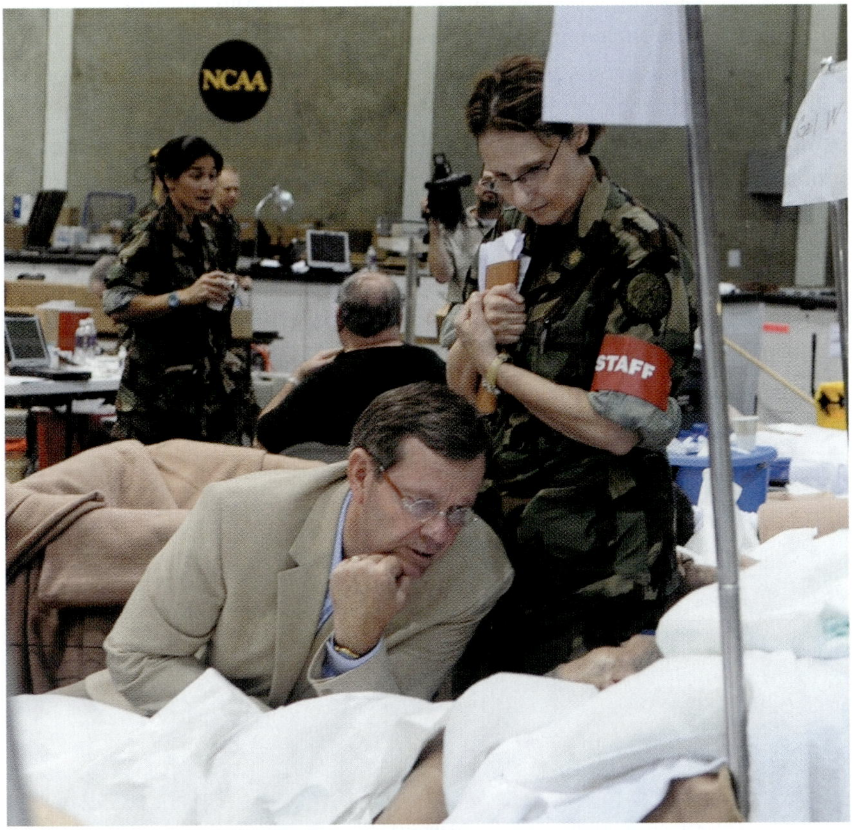

In the wake of Hurricane Gustav (2008), the then secretary of the federal Department of Health and Human Services, Michael Levitt, visits evacuees at the medical shelter, which had been set up at Louisiana State University in the Pete Maravich Assembly Center.

Staffing for Medical Shelters

Medical shelters are ideally staffed with a multidisciplinary team of medical personnel, but often because of limited funds have only nurses on staff. To ensure that these shelters can be adequately staffed, communities may contract in advance for personnel with needed skills, such as the local EMS or Medical Reserve Corps team. Desired staffing may include emergency medical technicians (EMTs), respiratory care personnel, physicians, and nurses. Many support staff are also needed. Their duties include creating records, maintaining paperwork, and distributing food.

Patients are often asked to bring their own supplies and special food, if possible. They are required to bring their own caregiver. Their caregivers are expected to assume primary responsibility for personal care tasks, such as dressing, walking, assisting patients to the bathroom, personal hygiene, and feeding. The sheltered individuals or their caregivers are responsible for administering routine medications, changing dressings, and handling special equipment. This includes being responsible for managing the oxygen and equipment. The patients and caregivers are assisted as needed by healthcare professionals.

Medical shelters, however, vary widely in the number of staff members and type and amount of equipment provided, depending on the resources available. Some medical shelters are very simple, set up in a gym or large room, with cots and nurses walking around with medical carts. Not all medical shelters can provide the equipment necessary for dialysis or intubation. Patients who need such treatment may have to be hospitalized.

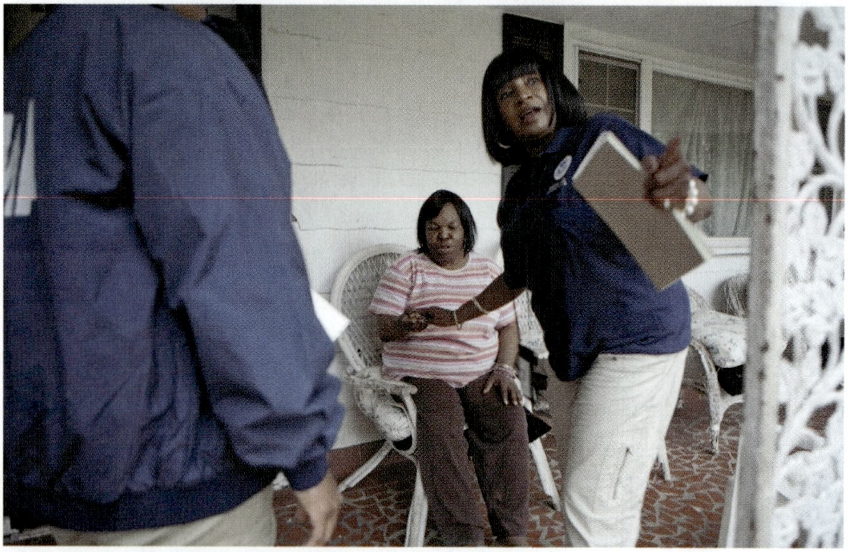

A community relations specialist discusses the options for disaster assistance and shelter with a blind resident in Chattanooga, Tennessee.

Communicating about Medical Shelters

State departments of health have procedures for educating the public about these specialized shelters and how to preregister for them, if needed. The public will be told:

- Who is eligible to go to the medical shelter
- What they should bring with them, such as necessary medical supplies and equipment, dietary foods, water, personal items such as eyeglasses, hygiene articles, and change of clothing

The plans for the medical shelter include procedures for the day-to-day running of the shelter and the conditions under which patients should be sent to hospitals. Arrangements may be made for the local EMS to transport residents from the shelter to a hospital.

Counseling Patients on Personal Medical Emergency Kits

As part of emergency and disaster preparedness, medical professionals should advise patients with chronic illnesses to pull together a medical emergency kit for evacuations. Each kit should contain a list of all medications the person takes and the dosages, insurance information, and medical records obtained from healthcare providers. (More information on nonmedical supplies for these personal evacuation and shelter-in-place kits is covered in Chapter 6.)

Each kit should also contain the type of medical supplies each person needs for a minimum of one week. For example, a person with diabetes should pack alcohol swabs, syringes, cotton balls, testing strips, blood glucose meters, a pen or pencil, and a pad of paper to record blood sugar levels. Patients should be prepared to store refrigerated medications in a cooler. They should always have a supply of frozen ice packs ready to go.

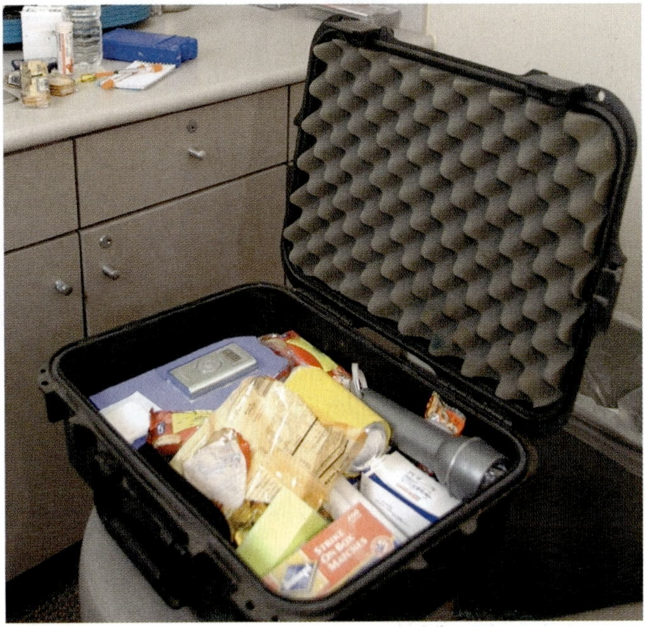

An emergency kit for someone diabetic might include (at a minimum) a glucose testing kit, snacks for stabilizing glucose, and a list of medications.

Patients should be encouraged to ask for a three-month supply when they fill their prescriptions, and refill them early so that they have enough medication in case a disaster strikes. Patients also need to check the expiration dates and use the stored medication before it expires and replace it with medication with a later expiration date. Parents should include their child's EIF in the emergency kit they prepare for children with chronic health conditions.

Patients should inspect their kits at least once a year. They should update insurance information, medication, and medical records, packing them in a waterproof plastic bag to prevent water damage. Patients will also want to keep a list of their healthcare providers and contact information. The emergency kit should be portable and should be stored in a place where it can be easily accessed. Family, friends, and neighbors of the patient should know where the emergency kit is kept.

Maintaining Electrical Medical Equipment

Patients who depend on equipment that requires electricity, such as ventilators, are particularly at risk during power outages. Advise these patients to plan ahead and do the following to be prepared:

- Notify their electric company, fire department, or EMS that they have a medical device that needs power.
- Check user instructions or call the distributor or manufacturer to find out whether the device can be used with batteries or a generator.
- Locate and hook up a generator, if possible.

When the power is restored following a disaster where electricity is down, check to be sure that the settings on the medical device have not changed during the power outage. Medical devices often reset themselves automatically to default settings when power is interrupted, as do digital clocks, and they need to be reset to the patient's personal requirements. Also, as area power networks are restored, voltage levels may fluctuate. This may cause devices to continue to reset or operate improperly. Be sure that patients have surge protectors on their electrical outlets and power strips for their medical devices.

If electronic devices are exposed to water or high levels of humidity, they also may not operate properly. Before using such a device, patients should do the following:

- Immediately turn off the power at the main circuit breaker if electrical circuits and equipment have gotten wet.
- Dry the device thoroughly. Wipe the outside of the device with a dry cloth.

A Closer Look

Emergency Generators

Homes, shelters, and healthcare facilities often rely on emergency generators to provide power for medical equipment during a power outage. In past disasters, failures to provide uninterrupted power were the result of lack of maintenance of the equipment before the storm. Most generator failures occurred because the generators had to operate continuously for an extended time.

Well-maintained generators are an important part of emergency and disaster preparedness. The following procedures must be followed to prevent carbon monoxide poisoning from generators:

- Never run a generator or a kerosene, natural gas, or gasoline-powered engine inside an enclosed structure, even if the doors or windows are open, unless the equipment is professionally installed and vented.
- Never run a generator or a gasoline-powered engine outside an open window or door where exhaust can waft into an enclosed area.

- Check devices for visible contamination.
- Check all power cords to be sure that they are not wet or damaged by water. If they are damaged, do not plug them into an electrical outlet.
- Check all settings and alarms to be sure they are working properly.
- Run quality control checks often to be sure that the device is performing accurately.

Handling a Medical Surge

After a disaster, healthcare facilities should expect and prepare for a high number of chronically ill patients needing treatment for their conditions. This is true not only for hospitals, but also for pharmacies, private medical practices, dialysis centers, and other facilities. During the disaster, patients' conditions may have worsened. These patients often need:

- Prescription medications, medical devices, and treatment such as dialysis
- Medical supplies, such as compression stockings, glucose testing supplies, or wheelchairs
- They may also need behavioral health services.

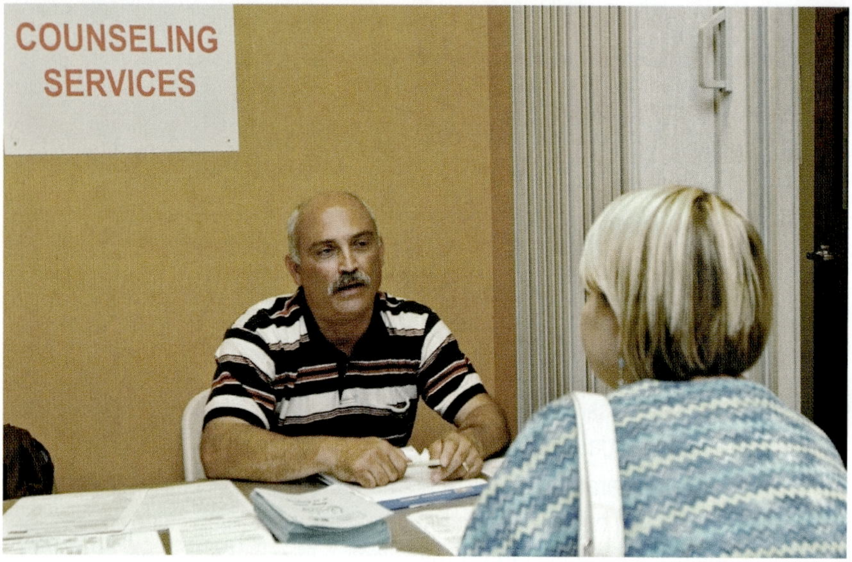

In Findlay, Ohio, a counselor talks with a patient whose home was damaged from flooding. Counseling desks, like this one, were staffed by a behavioral health organization at each of the Disaster Recovery Centers in the areas harmed by the massive flash flooding in the Midwest in August 2007.

Behavioral Health Services

During and after an emergency or disaster, those who have experienced the incident can become emotionally upset. Depending on the nature of the incident, these victims may have had their homes damaged or destroyed, and some may have even lost family members or friends. These losses can cause victims to feel stressed, anxious, or depressed, or even have more severe psychological symptoms. As noted earlier, victims of a disaster may express their worries, anger, and frustration to health professionals.

Providing Psychological First Aid

People often feel better just by talking about the experience and having someone listen carefully and affirm their feelings.

As a healthcare professional, you may listen to people share their disaster experiences to help them resolve their problems. The skills of empathetic listening are ones that health professionals can use in emergency and disaster response and in their everyday practice.

In the aftermath of an emergency or disaster, people often feel better just by talking about the experience. One technique to help people deal with their feelings is **Psychological First Aid**, which includes empathetic listening. A Closer Look provides tips for effective listening.

A Closer Look

Empathetic Listening Tips

In emergencies or disasters, good listening skills are essential when talking to victims or patients. Here are some tips for effective listening:

- Establish eye contact with patients.
- Do not judge what patients are saying.
- Allow silence. Just "being with" the survivors and their experience is supportive. Head nodding, caring facial expressions, and occasional "uh-huhs" let patients know that you are listening.
- Paraphrase what you have heard.
- Allow patients to express their emotions, which is an important part of healing. Let the victims know that it is okay to feel what they are feeling.

When responding to people, some people say things that they think are helpful but can sound judgmental or dismissive of their feelings. Do not say:

- "It could have been worse."
- "You can always get another car/house."
- "It's best if you just stay busy."
- "I know just how you feel."
- "You need to get on with your life."

To show that you are listening and care about people's experiences, you can say:

- "These are normal reactions to a disaster."
- "It is understandable that you feel this way."
- "It wasn't your fault. You did the best you could."
- "Things may never be the same, but they will get better, and you will feel better."

Behavioral Health Referrals

Although you can be helpful to patients through listening, patients may need help from behavioral health professionals. Allied health professionals are not trained to provide the type of counseling that is provided by a behavioral health professional. You need to know when, where, and how to refer patients to other resources. **Behavioral health providers**, also known as mental health professionals, have a key role in helping people who have survived a disaster. They are trained to provide both support and counseling services. Their work occurs immediately after the disaster and through the months or years that follow.

Behavioral health professionals in a community may mobilize and set up counseling programs at assistance centers or shelters, and at the locations where behavioral health services are usually provided. Counseling services are always provided by local or regional providers, and the federal government sends teams in only when the local capacity is not enough.

> **Expand Your Knowledge**
>
> SAMHSA provides a quarterly online newsletter for disaster behavioral health coordinators, local service providers, federal agencies, and nongovernmental organizations called *The Dialogue*. To read it, go to: **http:// EmDPrp2. ParadigmEducation.com/ dialogue**.

Within the US Department of Health and Human Services, there is an agency devoted to supporting behavioral health—the **Substance Abuse and Mental Health Services Administration (SAMHSA)**. SAMHSA hosts the **Disaster Technical Assistance Center (DTAC)** that provides a centralized site to guide disaster management planners and response personnel in organizing effective behavioral health services. Go to: **http://EmDPrp2 .ParadigmEducation.com/DCAT**.

When considering referring someone to counseling services, speak to your supervisor to find out who might be able to help and what resources are available. Tell your supervisor about patients who display these behaviors:

- Seeming disoriented—cannot remember things such as the date or time, do not know where they are, cannot recall events of the past 24 hours or understand what is happening
- Hearing, seeing, or thinking about things that are not real
- Not caring for themselves—not eating, bathing, or putting on clothes; unable to manage activities of daily living
- Having suicidal or homicidal thoughts or plans
- Abusing alcohol or drugs
- Being abused

Animal Care Services

Humans are not the only ones needing care and attention during a disaster. Many evacuation shelters cannot accept pets. However, shelters do allow people with **service animals**, or animals that are individually trained to do work or perform tasks for people with disabilities.

Dogs are the most common service animal. The Americans with Disabilities Act requires that dogs who are service animals be allowed to accompany their owners into shelters. Service animals can guide people who are blind, alert people who are deaf, pull wheelchairs, and remind a person with mental illness to take prescribed medications, among other tasks.

Pets often must be cared for through other arrangements. Pet owners are advised not to leave animals loose to fend for themselves, as they can quickly be in danger or cause danger to others. They can get in fights with other animals or possibly bite people, causing serious harm.

Owners should never leave animals chained up or caged outdoors where they can't escape flooding. They should be brought to an animal shelter that is not located in the evacuation zone. If there are no other options, it is best to leave the pets in a safe place in the home, with food and plenty of water. A note should be placed on the door and upper windows noting the presence of the animals and information about how the owners can be reached. This should be done even if the phones and Internet are not working, as this information will be useful when communications are restored. All animals should also have license and identification tags.

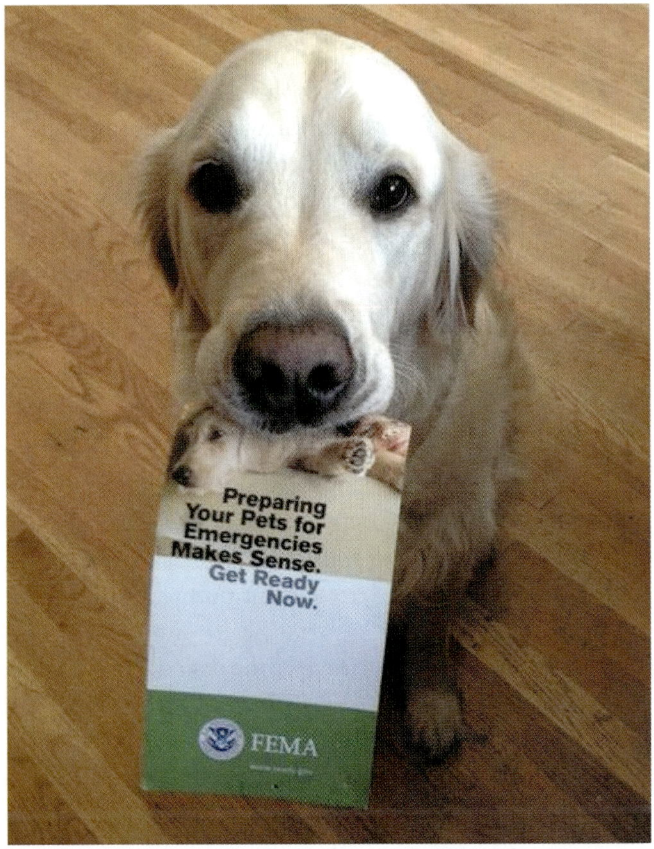

This FEMA image helps encourage pet owners to make a plan for their animals.

Animal Care Response and Recovery

Like other organizations, animal shelters need to have emergency and disaster plans, and they are likely to ask their regular volunteers and others to help them evacuate or address the needs of the many injured or ill animals in a disaster. The **National Animal Care & Control Association (NACA)** is a professional organization for animal shelters and animal welfare workers. NACA maintains a disaster database of those willing to assist at shelters and in animal rescue and care. For instance, after tornadoes struck in Moore, Oklahoma, NACA used the database to contact a woman from the Plattsmouth Police Department in Nebraska, which was six and a half hours away by car, to assist in the rescue and trapping of dangerous animals.

Veterinarians and veterinary technicians are essential in emergency and disaster response. Many volunteer in their communities and at their local animal shelters. Some serve as part of the **National Disaster Animal Response and Recovery Teams (NDARRTs)**. There are volunteer teams, organized and trained through The Humane Society of the United States, in all 50 states. They are dedicated to helping reunite lost and found animals with their owners. Besides their Humane Society training, NDARRT members are required to take certain FEMA courses (such as on the National Response Framework and National Incident Management System) for certification. Community Emergency Response Teams (CERTs) can also take course modules on animal response training.

A **Veterinary Medical Assistant Team (VMAT)** serves as the first responder for animals. The American Veterinary Medical Association (AVMA) organizes VMATs during emergencies and disasters. States may call in these teams to provide training on preparedness to veterinary medical professionals, shelters, zoos, farmers and ranchers, and others.

In the midst of or after a national disaster, the Assistant Secretary for Preparedness and Response may deploy its National Veterinary Response Team (NVRT), as part of the NDMS. The NVRT members work with the local animal shelters and rescue teams to treat injured and ill animals and to prevent outbreaks of any animal diseases. Members of the NVRT also provide health support for the working animals during the disaster response (such as the dogs and horses used for search and rescue and law enforcement).

Expand Your Knowledge

The Department of Homeland Security urges all pet owners to make emergency plans for their pets. For more information, go to: https://www.ready.gov/animals.

The Humane Society of the United States also provides guidance at: http://EmDPrp2.ParadigmEducation.com/HS-animal-prep.

Expand Your Knowledge

The American Veterinary Medical Association offers training opportunities to prepare for disasters at: http://EmDPrp2.ParadigmEducation.com/AVMA-training.

Chapter Summary

Many individuals are at particular risk during emergencies and disasters. The elderly, people with disabilities, and those who cannot care for themselves, such as unattended children, have special needs that must be addressed during emergency situations. Healthcare professionals need to know how to attend to these different populations.

Healthcare professionals need to know what advice to give people with chronic illnesses so that they can be prepared to deal with disasters. Those with chronic medical conditions should prepare emergency kits containing their medications and medical supplies. Individuals with medical conditions that require more complex care or who have serious medical conditions that cannot be properly cared for in the evacuation shelters set up for the general population, should be advised to seek a medical shelter.

Disaster victims may also experience psychological or emotional stress. Healthcare professionals can be helpful by acknowledging the difficulties that their patients are experiencing. They need to know the skills of empathetic listening and response, and the signs of a patient needing a referral to a behavioral health specialist.

In addition, health professionals should tell their patients that they cannot bring pets into general evacuation shelters. They can refer patients to the local and national organizations that support the care and rescue of pets following an emergency or disaster.

Additional Resources

To extend the content presented in this chapter, take advantage of the resources available through the chapter's eBook resource links and the end-of-chapter link. These resources include informational supplements and flash cards for terms and abbreviations.

Key Terms	
at-risk populations	psychological first aid
behavioral health provider	reunification
continuity of care	service animals
emergency information form	shelf life
medical shelter	

Recognizing Terms

Choose the word or phrase from the list of key terms that best matches each of the following descriptions. Your instructor may ask you to submit your work for grading or may provide you with an answer key for self-assessment.

1. Period of time in which a medication is viable __________
2. Facilities outfitted with equipment and staff to care for patients who cannot be cared for in general shelters __________
3. Groups, such as the elderly, people with disabilities, children, and people who do not speak English, that have special healthcare needs during and after a disaster __________
4. A document that summarizes the medical condition, medications, and other medical needs of children with chronic medical conditions __________
5. Bringing loved ones who have been separated back together __________
6. A type of mental health professional who helps people deal with the experience of a disaster __________
7. Dogs that are individually trained to do work or perform tasks for people with disabilities __________

Reviewing Concepts

Choose the response that best answers the question or completes the sentence. Your instructor may ask you to submit your work for grading or may provide you with an answer key for self-assessment.

1. An example of a chronic disease is
   a. the common cold.
   b. influenza.
   c. a broken bone.
   d. asthma.
2. During an emergency, all of the following would be considered patients with special needs except people who need
   a. corrective lenses.
   b. skilled nursing but not hospitalization.
   c. their vital signs monitored.
   d. professional medical observation.

3. An emergency medical kit should contain which of the following? (Select all that apply.)
   a. a medical ID bracelet
   b. at least a week's supply of medical supplies
   c. a list of healthcare providers
   d. a list of the medications
4. Who has responsibility for setting up medical shelters?
   a. the federal government
   b. the state health department
   c. the American Red Cross
   d. private healthcare contractors
5. An essential piece of equipment for medical shelters is a
   a. defibrillator.
   b. ventilator.
   c. refrigerator.
   d. generator.
6. What type of pets are allowed in shelters?
   a. small animals
   b. animals that need food and water
   c. service animals
   d. dogs that are sick
7. What specialized training do members of the National Veterinary Response Teams receive to prepare them to respond in a disaster? (Select all that apply.)
   a. Humane Society courses
   b. FEMA courses
   c. Red Cross courses
   d. courses on the Internet
8. Which of the following techniques are used in psychological first aid? (Select all that apply.)
   a. Establish eye contact with patients.
   b. Judge and repeat back what patients are saying.
   c. Make sure the person talks all the time.
   d. Nod your head, use caring facial expressions, and occasionally say "uh-huhs."
   e. Paraphrase what you have heard.

9. What does the Emergency Prescription Assistance Program do?
   a. Coordinate with pharmacies during an emergency.
   b. Provide the medical history of people who have been in a disaster.
   c. Provide a 30-day supply of prescription medications, specific medical supplies, vaccines, and certain medical equipment.
   d. Stockpile medications and medical supplies.

10. Which group helps owners and pets reunite after a disaster?
    a. FEMA
    b. NDMS
    c. NDARRT
    d. CDC

Exploring Emergency Preparedness Issues

Complete the following activities to further explore the concepts found in this chapter. Your instructor may ask you to submit your work for grading or may provide you with guidance for self-assessment.

1. Identify the groups of patients cared for by your health profession who could be defined as "at risk" in the event of a disaster. Describe their special needs during a disaster. What would happen to their care if there was no power and/or no safe water or food? What resources would these patients need? Which agencies in the community could be helpful in planning to care for these patients? What plans would need to be developed in advance to reach out to your patients? What services could your profession offer? Summarize your response in a two-page report.

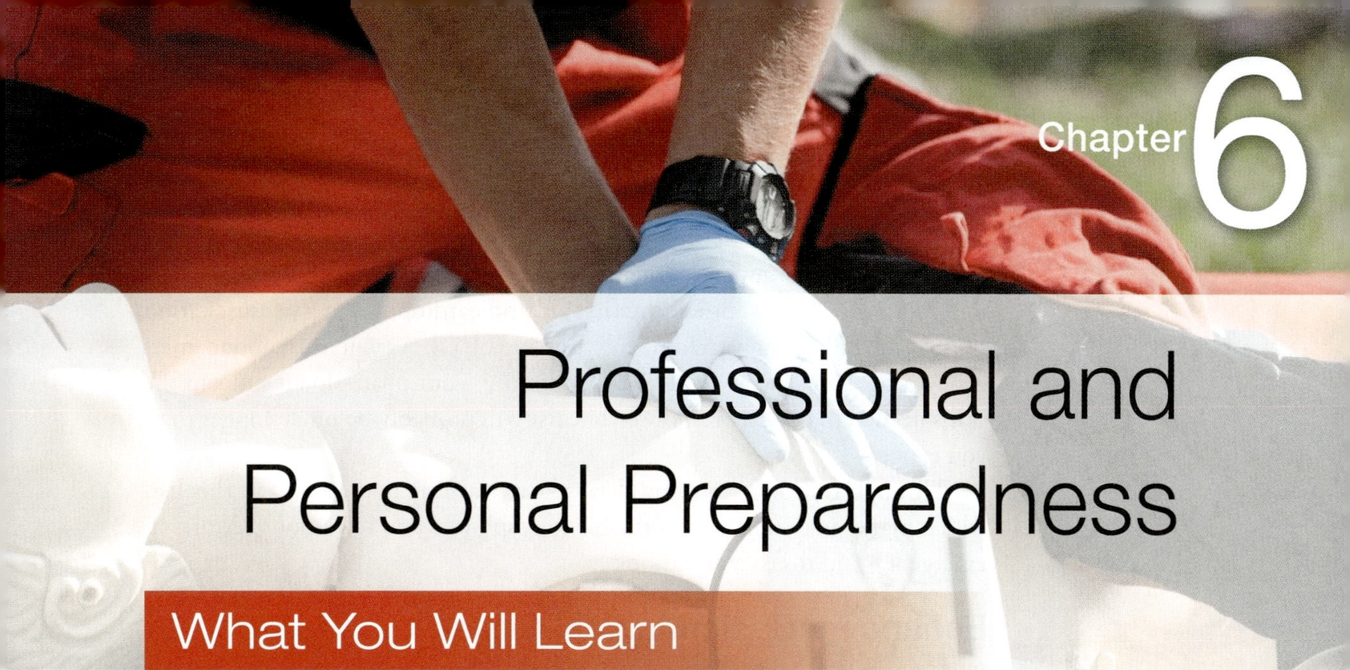

Chapter 6

Professional and Personal Preparedness

What You Will Learn

- What you need to know and how you can apply your professional skills to emergency and disaster situations
- Ways to enhance your basic medical skills
- Your role in your employer's emergency action plan and disaster training procedures
- What is entailed in volunteering for emergency and disaster work
- How to recognize the sources and signs of stress and learn how to cope with stress
- How to help yourself, your family, and your neighborhood prepare

Emergency and disaster preparedness is for everyone, including government agencies, businesses, healthcare facilities, and other organizations in the community. It is also for you, as a health professional and as a citizen. You can prepare for your part in emergency and disaster preparedness and response by developing appropriate skills, learning the emergency plan of your employer, exploring volunteer opportunities, finding ways to cope with the stress of response work, and preparing your family and neighborhood for whatever may happen.

Sharpening Your Response Skills

As an allied health professional, you have many clinical and administrative skills that are invaluable in emergency and disaster responses. These skills may include interviewing patients for their medical and medication histories, taking vital signs, providing first aid and cardiopulmonary resuscitation (CPR), administering vaccines, and drawing blood. As you learn about emergency procedures, keep an "I can" list, linking your professional skills to the skills needed in disaster response. The list will probably be much longer than you expect!

Through training, you can always keep learning and adding to this list, which makes you even more valuable to employers and to response efforts in emergency and disaster situations.

Enhancing Basic Medical Skills

When healthcare systems are disabled or destroyed, it will be difficult to provide services, especially during a medical surge. To meet this increased demand, communities will rely on the availability and support of individuals with basic medical skills. Enrolling in continuing education courses and earning additional certifications that enhance your medical skills can enrich your professional résumé and job opportunities while expanding your ability to provide needed medical services in a disaster.

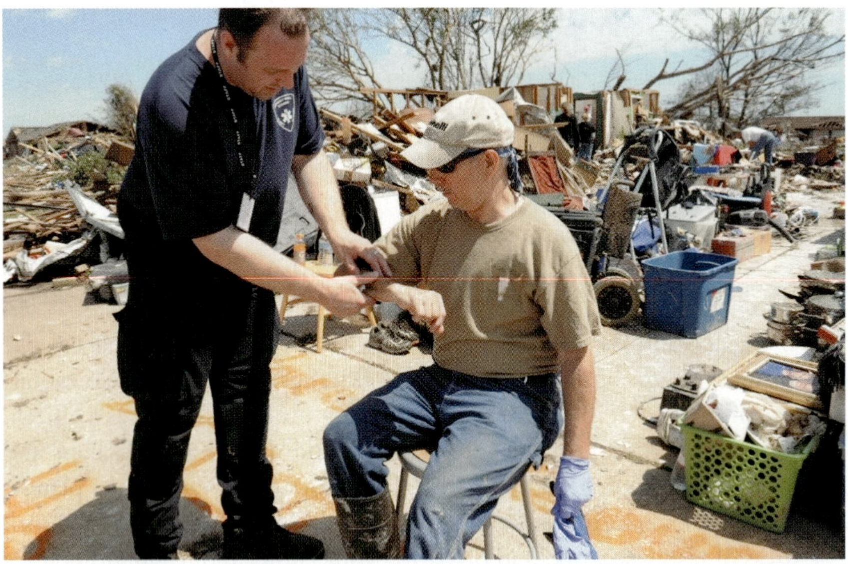

A local resident of Moore, Oklahoma, receives medical attention from a disaster volunteer after the tornado on May 20, 2013.

Key Acronyms	
BLS	basic life support
CPR	cardiopulmonary resuscitation
ECC	emergency cardiovascular care
EMAC	Emergency Management Assistance Compact
ESAR-VHP	Emergency System for Advance Registration of Volunteer Health Professionals

First Aid Imagine that you are the first person to arrive at the scene of an emergency and people are injured. Would you be able to provide first aid until more help arrived? First aid is a collection of initial responses to injuries that are simple, potentially lifesaving medical techniques delivered with minimal or no medical equipment. Providing first aid is something that everyone can do with the right training.

Training in first aid techniques includes how to decide the priorities, manage the emergency, and treat the following:

- minor bleeding and minor burns
- choking, fainting, bites and stings, sprains and strains
- an unresponsive victim

Professionals providing first aid also learn how to communicate with the patient and others at the incident site and how to get appropriate assistance.

First aid training is part of most educational programs in allied health. Many healthcare organizations require that healthcare professionals maintain their certification in first aid by taking courses. Many hospitals offer first aid courses. Local chapters of the American Red Cross also teach a variety of first aid and medical response courses. Some of their courses can be partially completed online. You can then work in person with a Red Cross instructor to practice and polish your skills.

Cardiopulmonary Resuscitation **Cardiopulmonary resuscitation (CPR)** is a step-by-step process used to restart the beating of a heart and breathing when both have ceased. CPR involves four steps: contract chest in comprehensions, clear airways, give breath, and repeat. By getting trained to perform CPR, you can help someone in distress when other bystanders may not know this lifesaving skill.

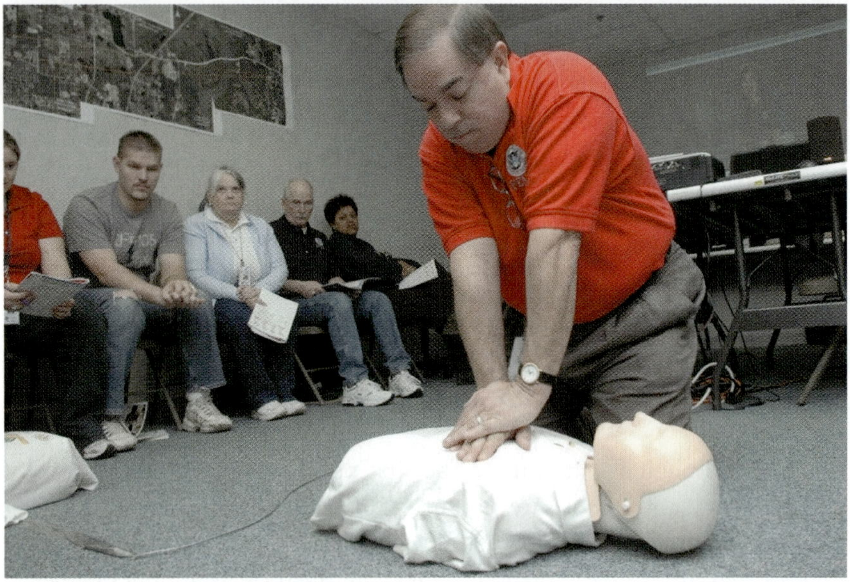

Here, CPR techniques are being demonstrated in an American Red Cross training class.

Emergency Cardiovascular Care **Emergency cardiovascular care (ECC)** is a higher-level skill that requires special training. You will learn techniques for adult, pediatric, and CPR conducted by two people; clearing an obstructed airway; and properly applying an automated external defibrillator (AED) or mask.

Basic Life Support **Basic life support (BLS)** requires additional training and certification that includes ECC and added skills of critical thinking, problem solving, communication, and being part of an emergency medical team. BLS training includes learning about safety and infection control procedures and legal considerations. Allied health professionals and civilians from all backgrounds can get trained in BLS. Classes for CPR, ECC, and BLS are offered through the American Red Cross, the American Heart Association, and many hospitals and allied health programs. Once certified, practice these skills often to maintain them.

Preparing to Work without Technology

In thinking about being prepared at your work for an emergency or disaster, one of the questions you should consider is: could you perform the essential tasks of your job without the technology that you use everyday? You would need to know this answer if the power goes out and backup power fails. Computers, intravenous (IV) pumps, and respirators require electricity to operate. Learning how to use hand-powered equipment and processes and other low-tech ways to perform core tasks is an important part of emergency and disaster preparedness for all health professionals.

Instructors and professionals who have been in their fields for many years may know how the work was done before currrent technology. If you work with seasoned professionals, ask them to help you learn what to do. They may be able to teach you how to work without technology.

Providing Support Services

Allied health professionals can also fill many support roles in disaster response because of their experience in working with patients and the health-care system. When there are many patients and little time, support workers are critical to being able to deliver the increased need of services to so many patients. As demonstrated in Chapter 4, at the Point of Dispensing sites,

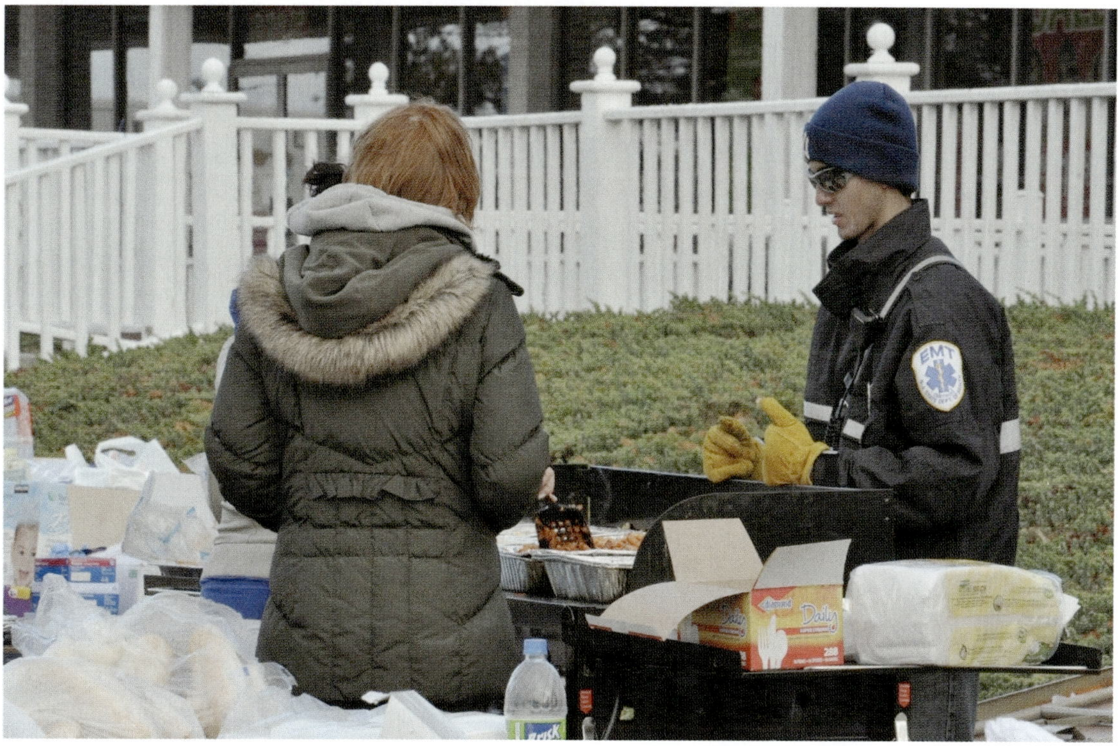

An EMT at a Point of Distribution site in Wall Township, New Jersey, offers hot food to a Hurricane Sandy survivor November 3, 2012.

additional workers are needed to help unpack, organize, and maintain stores of medicines and supplies; direct patients; provide communications links; translate; control crowds; and more. Allied health workers are also helpful in support positions at evacuation shelters and Point of Distribution centers for food and water and other disaster supplies.

Support work takes many forms. For example, in 2001 in the hours that followed the attack of the World Trade Center, hospitals activated their emergency operations plans. At White Plains Hospital, which was 30 miles north, sonographers (ultrasound specialists) were asked to prepare rooms so that families of victims who lived nearby could view the bodies. The sonographers cleared rooms, got gurneys ready, and had food and drink available for families. This work was important to the families and the medical facility.

Participating in Facility Preparedness

OSHA requires that all companies with more than 10 employees, including those in healthcare, such as pharmacies, have a written **emergency action plan**.

Most companies and businesses explain the emergency plan through orientation sessions for new employees, departmental staff meetings, emergency exercises, and in the employer's policy manual. The plan should include the

A Closer Look

A Facility Emergency Action Plan

A facility emergency action plan should identify and explain the actions to be taken in an emergency or disaster. A good emergency plan:

- Identifies potential threats and hazards
- Identifies emergency response and reporting procedures
- Defines roles and expectations of employees
- Describes procedures for warnings and communication
- Identifies the location and proper use of emergency equipment
- Describes building and equipment shutdown procedures
- Identifies evacuation procedures and rendezvous places
- Provides exit maps or diagrams
- Explains how all personnel, visitors, and patients will be accounted for
- Describes procedures for sheltering in the facility
- Identifies rescue and medical tasks
- Provides guidelines and timelines for training and drills

tasks assigned to your department, identify which staff members will be responsible for each task in various types of emergencies, and state how the tasks are to be accomplished. For example, if your work area contains special hazards, such as flammable or radioactive materials, you may be responsible for securing these materials in an emergency.

The plan will also explain how you will be notified when an emergency or disaster has occurred. Besides the facility emergency alert, there should be a plan for contacting employees who are not on duty.

The plan must also include emergency exercises. As with hospitals and medical clinics, these mock disaster drills allow you and the rest of the staff to practice the facility plan and put your skills into action.

You will need to know evacuation procedures and the location of the preassigned gathering places in the facility in case of a tornado, earthquake, flood, or other event. You may also receive training in emergency procedures or available equipment, such as fire extinguishers.

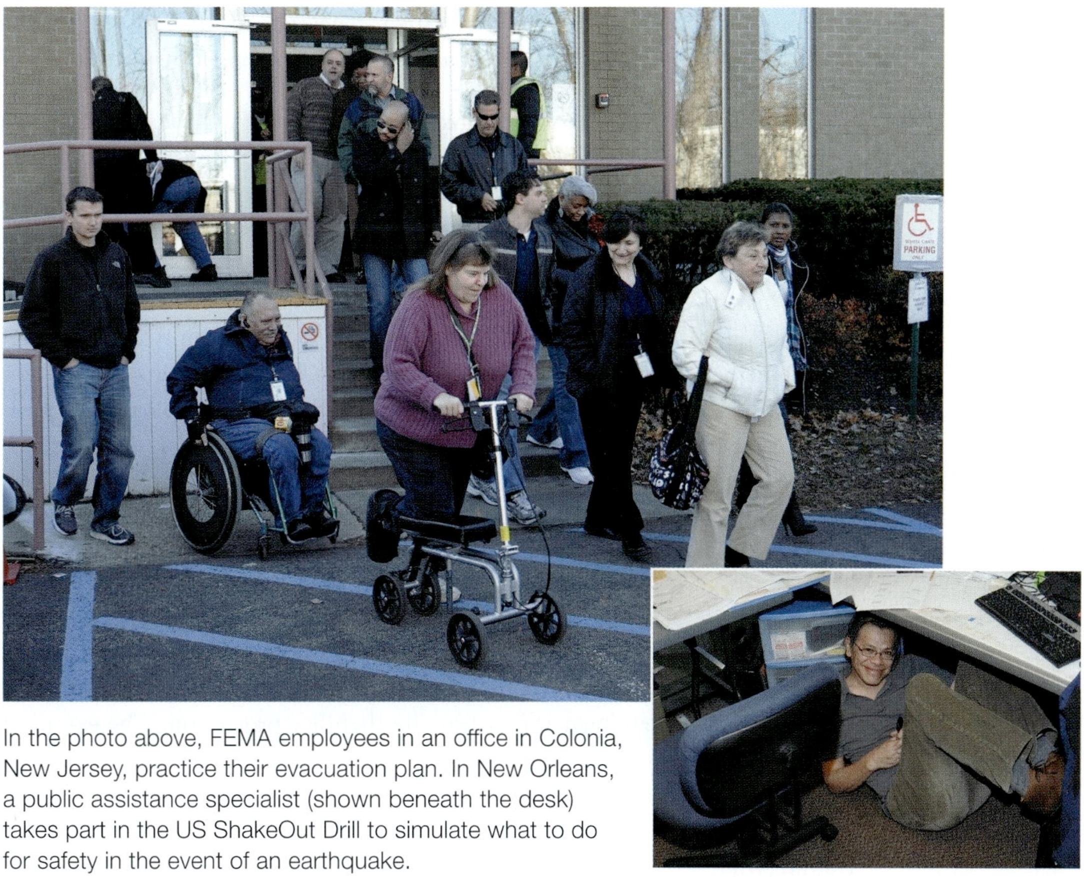

In the photo above, FEMA employees in an office in Colonia, New Jersey, practice their evacuation plan. In New Orleans, a public assistance specialist (shown beneath the desk) takes part in the US ShakeOut Drill to simulate what to do for safety in the event of an earthquake.

How to Volunteer

In addition to any workplace responses, you may want to volunteer your professional services on a medical response team. Allied health professionals can get involved in many ways. During the response to Hurricane Sandy in 2012, over 2,300 healthcare workers were deployed from the National Disaster Medical System and US Public Health Service Commissioned Corps. They cared for more than 6,700 residents at overwhelmed hospitals and at shelters in New York and New Jersey. These volunteers made a real difference for patients and communities, and you can too.

Preregistration for Credentialing and Efficiency

When a disaster takes place, most allied health professionals are eager to help. To be most effective, it is best to register in advance. By doing this, you join an organized preparedness effort. You will know details of how the volunteer organization plans to help and the types of tasks it might perform in a disaster. Preregistered medical volunteers generally receive training and are assigned to a team that has access to equipment and supplies to support the team's needs.

Credentialing When you preregister, organizations will be able to verify your credentials so that you can be ready to work when a disaster occurs. This process will include a verification of the volunteer's identity, license, training, skills, and competencies. Many state's require licenses in order to practice your profession. Having a license is an important credential because it demonstrates that the licensee has achieved a level of education, training and skills. Your credentials will determine which tasks you will be permitted to perform in an emergency and disaster. Only those who are registered in advance can be sure that their credentials will be verified in time for them to use their skills when and where they are needed.

If you are preregistered and credentialed to volunteer with an organization that sends volunteers out of state, then your licensure, certification, and credentialing may be temporarily transferred to another state where a disaster has been declared. Otherwise, you may not be permitted to work in a different state.

Liability Another reason that preregistration and credentialing are important is that, to be protected when providing response services, volunteers must be registered with an agency that provides liability protection. The extent of the liability coverage depends on the organization that deploys the volunteers.

Many health professionals are covered by their employer and do not have independent coverage for malpractice. This coverage may not cover you when volunteering, so you will need to ask about malpractice coverage when you register to volunteer.

It is helpful to know your state's **Good Samaritan laws**. These are laws that provide legal protection for individuals helping people who are injured. Does your state have statutes that provide protection to those performing emergency care during a disaster? Additionally, if you have professional liability insurance coverage, determine whether the coverage is effective if you work outside your usual practice settings.

If you have not had the chance to preregister, then contact a local response organization and offer your services and let them know your position, training, and credentials. Group leaders who organize volunteers will want to know the skills of each volunteer. Find out if the liability insurance of the organization covers the volunteers working within their scope of practice.

Be Aware

When volunteering, do not bring along medical supplies, clothing, or food for the victims, unless you've been instructed to do so ahead of time. Donated supplies may not be used (or needed) if not requested and part of a distribution system.

Where to Register for Healthcare Volunteering

Each state has an **Emergency System for the Advance Registration of Volunteer Health Professionals (ESAR-VHP)**. These systems are designed to assess and preregister volunteer health professionals for work both within their own and in other states during public health and other emergencies. The Assistant Secretary for Preparedness and Response oversees the ESAR-VHP. The states work with the ESAR-VHP to develop a preregistration program to allow for swift activation of certified healthcare volunteers when an emergency or disaster is predicted or occurs.

Each state-based system contains readily available, verifiable, current information about the identity, licensing, and credentials of each volunteer. When the governor calls a state of emergency, these preregistered volunteers are ready to serve. To begin the process of registering, you can find your state and profession on the web page for the ESAR-VHP at: **http://EmDPrp2.ParadigmEducation.com/esar-vhp-register**.

Heroes Corner

Volunteer Power

Over 11,000 volunteers participated in more than 80 service projects to help communities and individuals clean up after Hurricane Sandy through NYC Service, a division of the mayor's office that organizes volunteers and donated resources.

One organization that responded to the call of NYC Service, Respond & Rebuild, organized hundreds of citizen volunteers in the Rockaway area within 24 hours after the storm passed. They have trained volunteers, even establishing field team leadership internships. Volunteers removed rotting debris, dried out rooms, and removed mold that grew in flooded homes. They cleaned over 100 structures so residents could move back into their homes. The organization estimates that in the aftermath and years after Sandy, it logged over 40,000 hours, worked on more than 400 homes, and supplied more than $800,000 in free services.

People who preregister with the ESAR-VHP may also be deployed by the governor to other states through the **Emergency Management Assistance Compact (EMAC)**. EMAC is a mutual aid agreement that facilitates the sharing of resources, personnel, and equipment across state lines during disasters. It covers all states, the District of Columbia, Puerto Rico, and the US Virgin Islands. During the 2011 response to Hurricane Irene and Tropical Storm Lee, 10 states requested EMAC assistance. Twenty-five states provided over 1,100 personnel.

If you want to volunteer to serve in your own community, contact your municipal and county offices of emergency management or health departments. You will be directed to the person who handles the recruitment of volunteers. You can also preregister to be part of a DMAT, MRC, CERT, or one of the other active response groups described in Chapter 2. (See "A Closer Look" on the next page.)

Also, at the time of disaster, local service groups, such as the Rotary and Lions Clubs, play key roles in providing support and volunteers. If you have not preregistered and a disaster strikes your community, you could volunteer with one of these groups. To choose one that fits you, check in with local organizations or explore those posted on the US Chamber of Commerce web page at: **http:/EmDPrp2.ParadigmEducation.com/USChamber-list.**

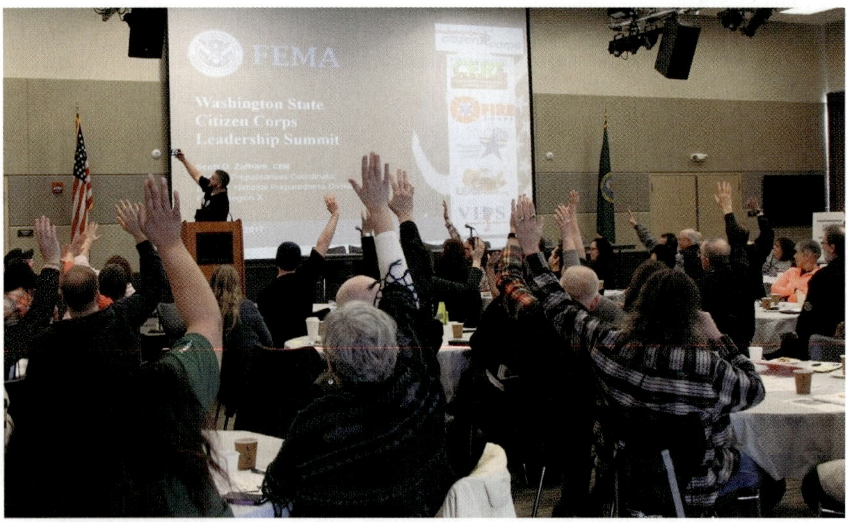

At a Washington State Citizen Corps Leadership Summit for Disaster Preparedness in 2017, participants willing to volunteer raised their hands. Summit attendees included members of the Medical Reserve Corps, Community Emergency Response Teams, local nongovernmental organizations, and local/state/federal emergency management personnel.

A Closer Look

Register Now to Be Ready Later

These organizations encourage you to preregister and receive training. As healthcare professionals have unique and valuable skills, it is good to try to volunteer with groups providing healthcare services first. If that is not possible, there are other organizations where you could offer a hand.

National Disaster Medical System Teams

The rapid-response DMATs are state based but can be deployed around the country during a national disaster. To become part of a team, apply for the position through USAJobs.gov, using the search keyword "NDMS." For more information, go to: **http://EmDPrp2.ParadigmEducation.com/NDMS-register**.

Medical Reserve Corps

To serve within your community and region, preregister with the MRC, which coordinates with local communities and healthcare facilities. MRC unit leaders are asked to ensure that local community response needs are met before volunteers are deployed to assist outside the area. To locate the nearest unit in your state, go to **http://EmDPrp2.ParadigmEducation.com/MRC-register**.

Community Emergency Response Teams

With CERT, you will learn first response medical procedures, fire safety, search and rescue, and other basic disaster response skills. First you must receive your training from one of the federal training centers or an official sponsoring agency, such as the state office of emergency management, the fire department, or police department. Locate a program in your community by inserting your zip code in the CERT page or through the CERT website: **http://EmDPrp2.ParadigmEducation.com/CERT-registering**.

Team Rubicon

Team Rubicon begins by having you choose your state on its map to register, and you can list the kind of jobs you are interested in working on. It specifically recruits medical professionals for teams. Visit: **http://EmDPrp2.ParadigmEducation.com/TR-register**.

The American Red Cross

Many communities have local Red Cross chapters that train and organize volunteers. Volunteers can sign up to participate as part of disaster services to be deployed during major disasters. For current opportunities in disaster work, go to its disaster volunteer page: **http://EmDPrp2.ParadigmEducation.com/RCross-register**.

The Salvation Army Emergency Disaster Services

Volunteers provide food, emergency communications, disaster social services, management of donations, recovery programs, and emotional and spiritual care. You take classes to prepare. For training locations, dates, and course descriptions, find your state in the location finder at **http://disaster.salvationarmyusa.org/training/**.

FEMA Corps

The FEMA Corps experiences are internships in disaster planning and response work arranged with Americorps. You need to apply in advance to serve full time for a specific term. Go to: **http://EmDPrp2.ParadigmEducation.com/FEMAC-apply**.

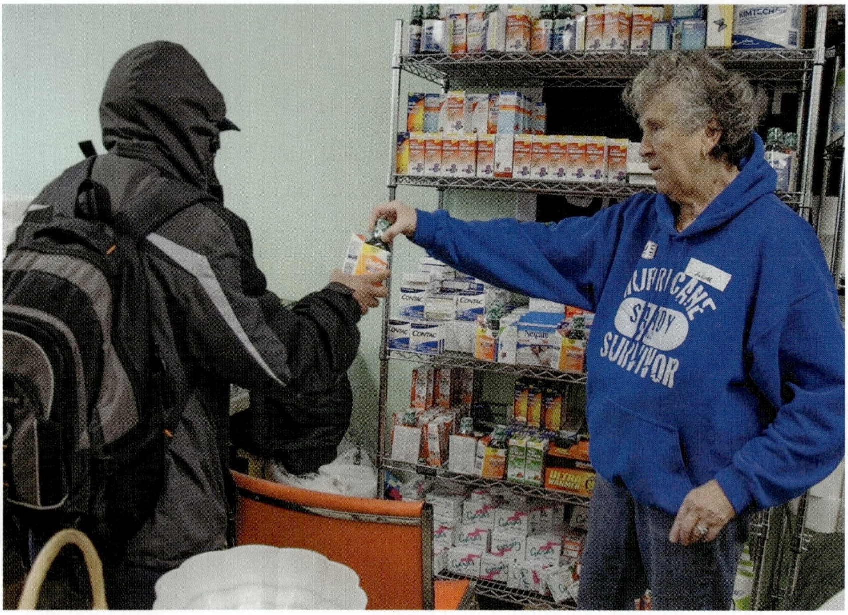

On January. 29, 2013, a local resident volunteer provides donated over-the-counter medications to a victim of Hurricane Sandy in Union Beach, New Jersey.

Just-in-Time Volunteer Training

For those who did not preregister but have volunteered, many emergency agencies and nonprofits have developed **just-in-time training** programs, which are specific last-minute training for tasks the volunteer will be performing at the response site. For example, a nurse might receive just-in-time training for a mass vaccination in response to a disease outbreak or a pharmacy technician might receive just-in-time training to help dispense medication.

When there are not enough pre-registered health professionals to meet the needs during a disaster, communities often make plans to recruit and incorporate volunteers. For example, retired healthcare clinicians may be contacted and asked to perform limited medical tasks. Nonclinical retirees and others may be asked to answer phones or direct patients.

Working Conditions at a Volunteer Site

Before volunteering to work in a disaster area, know what to expect. You might work on an established team or be assigned work in another hospital to support facility staff. Or you might also work at an alternative care site, evacuation shelter, Point of Dispensing site, or Point of Distribution center. If you are volunteering with a nongovernmental organization, you might find yourself helping with cleanup at an incident site or helping someone clean mold from the walls of his or her home.

A Closer Look

Expected Working Conditions

Health professionals who volunteer for a federal assignment in a disaster area should expect to:

- Work 12-hour shifts for two weeks or longer
- Be housed in tents, possibly with no showers, and sleep on bed rolls or cots
- Not have air-conditioning or heat
- Stand for long stretches of time
- Eat military ready-to-eat meals and food products
- Use portable toilets

Disaster areas usually have limited supplies of food, safe water, and medicine. As a volunteer, you may need current immunizations to protect against diseases, such as hepatitis B and tetanus. Workers often have long shifts with little rest, so physical stamina and good health are important considerations. You may also need transportation as well as specific clothing and equipment to work at affected sites.

Volunteers are expected to bring enough clothing, hygiene products, and so on for the expected period of service. During the recovery from Hurricane Sandy, electrical workers came from around the country to repair utility lines. When the workers arrived, the weather was mild, but it took months to rebuild the electrical lines, and the weather changed. Few workers had the proper clothing to work out of doors in the late fall and winter, so they had to purchase clothes.

Preparing for Stress

Besides being prepared for demanding physical conditions, volunteers must also be psychologically prepared. They will be caring for victims who may have lost family members and homes. Victims may have witnessed violence or suffering and may be feeling anguish, anger, and sadness. You must be able to provide support, even if you are experiencing many of the same emotions. Regardless of the emergency, whether you respond as an employee or volunteer, you will encounter situations that cause stress. Some sources of stress cannot be avoided, but there are many ways to reduce and cope with stress. Personal preparedness includes anticipating that you will experience stress and knowing how to deal with it.

Sources of Stress

Even with the best planning, situations may be chaotic. Health professionals may feel that no matter how much they do, it is not enough. Some victims will be grateful for the help they receive, whereas others may be angry at the situation and take their anger out on those who are helping them. Additionally, you may be a victim. Your home may be destroyed, or members of your family may be hurt or worse. It is normal and expected that people will experience stress under these circumstances. Even experienced emergency responders are affected.

On the positive side, many people find that working together for a common good brings them closer together. The experience can influence professional and personal beliefs or priorities and provide a deep sense of satisfaction about making an important contribution. Even if you have positive feelings about this service, expect the work to be difficult and stressful.

Recognizing Signs of Stress and Burnout

No one who sees or experiences a disaster can remain untouched by it. Although most healthcare professionals function well during and after a disaster, it is normal for them to feel stressed or saddened about what has happened—to them, the people they care about, and their community. You may feel angry, powerless, frightened, or guilty for surviving. These are normal reactions.

A Closer Look

Stress-Causing Situations

During a disaster, it is important to be alert to the many situations that can be stressful:

- You, your family, friends, or co-workers may be among the victims.
- Communications may be down, so it may not be clear what is happening.
- Supplies may be inadequate.
- Weather conditions may be extreme.
- Tasks are likely to be physically exhausting and/or dangerous.
- You may become sleep deprived.
- You may feel that you cannot do enough to help victims.
- You may witness suffering and death.
- There may be struggles over decision making and authority.
- The disaster may bring back painful memories of previous experiences.

During the response, everyone concentrates on helping the victims of the disaster. The needs of the workers may be initially ignored or seen as less important than those of the victims. As a disaster worker, you may not be prepared for your own emotional reactions to the situation.

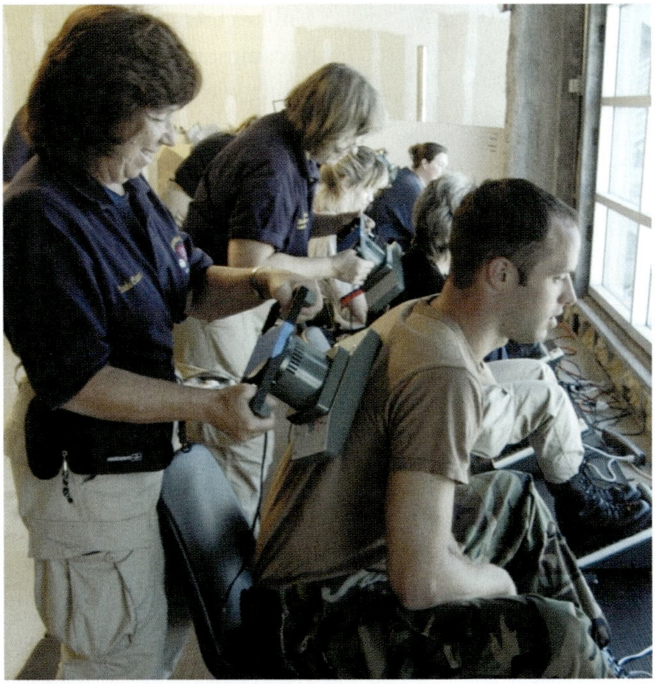

During Hurricane Katrina, behavioral health workers from a DMAT provided massages to relieve the stress of responders. While being massaged, the workers were encouraged to talk about their experiences during this response.

Sometimes stress builds up and leads to **burnout**, which is a condition of emotional exhaustion. This is something to watch for. Volunteers suffering from burnout may no longer feel enthusiastic about their work, they may work less efficiently, and they may feel tired even when they get enough sleep. They may be irritable about their jobs and toward their colleagues. Sometimes memories of the disaster intrude on their consciousness without warning. Stress may make people feel distant from those they are normally close to.

Some may pull away from family and friends. Often, stress will put a strain on personal relationships. Some people may try to cope with stress by using drugs or alcohol. Other warning signs include having difficulty concentrating or sleeping and a variety of physical symptoms, such as headaches, gastrointestinal problems, and a decrease in appetite or sexual desire. People experiencing burnout may drink too much coffee or alcohol, or smoke too much.

When workers suffer from burnout, they do not work as hard, which diminishes the efficiency of their team. They may put themselves in physical or emotional danger if they are not concentrating on what they are doing while working.

People who work in a disaster may face more stress when they return home. What they experienced in the field is different from their normal routine. When they return home, they may need time to adjust. However, their family will probably want their attention or help after their absence. Family members may be angry that the worker was gone, especially if they were also victims of the disaster and they were responding to the effects of the disaster on their own lives.

Expand Your Knowledge

The SAMHSA toll-free helpline was a valued resource for victims of disasters. The Disaster Distress Helpline is available at 800-985-5990 or text TalkWithUs to 666746. You can learn more at **http://EmDPrp2.ParadigmEducation.com/helpline**.

Unlike emergency workers, whose full-time job involves dealing with crises in the community, healthcare professionals often do not have much experience in dealing with disasters. It will help you to know in advance the ways you may react. Learn the signs of stress and burnout in yourself and your coworkers.

The federal Substance Abuse and Mental Health Services Administration (SAMHSA) offers a Disaster Distress Helpline for response workers. It is staffed by trained counselors for multilingual and confidential crisis counseling and references for follow-up care. You can also receive information on recognizing stress and coping tips at its website. Visit: **http://EmDPrp2.ParadigmEducation.com/SAMHSA-stress-tips.**

Ways to Cope

Part of the responsibility of protecting workers from stress belongs to those supervising the response. These managers should recognize and show appreciation for the important work being done. Understanding the toll this work can take on people, managers should arrange for adequate breaks during rescue and relief operations. They also should arrange for debriefing sessions at the appropriate times. These sessions provide an opportunity to discuss their experiences and share feelings.

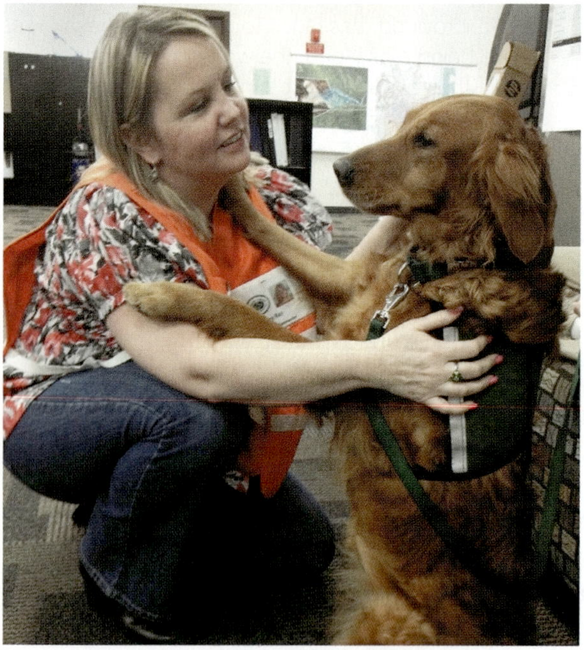

Responders benefit from relief from stress. Dog teams can be deployed to bring cheer and support to both victims and responders.

Organizations use different techniques with disaster workers to help them deal with stress. Opportunities to relieve stress are not usually offered alone but as part of an ongoing system of support in disaster situations. There are a number of approaches that can be used. Two of these include defusing and crisis intervention counseling.

- **Defusing** is a brief, informal procedure used after an event to help the disaster workers voice their concerns. In defusing, behavioral health professionals hold 10- to 30-minute sessions in which workers can express their thoughts and feelings about what they are doing and have encountered. Workers may need to talk about an unexpected incident, such as an accident; the discovery of an injured person; or a conflict between workers, with a supervisor, or with a victim. Disaster workers, like victims, should be able to talk about their experiences and feelings in both informal and formal settings. They are listened to with empathy and acceptance so that they defuse some of their feelings.

- **Crisis intervention counseling** uses a set of dialog techniques that help participants feel more in control during a crisis. In group or individual counseling, workers have an opportunity to share their feelings and help identify solutions to recover from the disaster. The counseling aims at promoting resilience, empowerment, and stress recovery. The counseling sessions also serve to identify any participants who could benefit from a referral to a behavioral health professional.

A Closer Look

Personal Tools for Handling Stress

You can use many techniques to reduce tension and anxiety during the response phase and in the weeks and months after you return home. Some of these techniques include:

- Recognize, understand, and appreciate your feelings. It is normal to have strong feelings and reactions.
- Be tolerant of the reactions of other relief workers and victims. Disasters are a time of stress for everyone. People may feel angry, shocked, or frightened. They may feel guilty because they are physically okay, whereas others are not. People who have gone through disasters feel grief, whether for people they know or for victims they do not know. They may feel despair and a sense of helplessness. They may also seem irritable and short-tempered.
- Try relaxation techniques involving breathing, positive thinking, yoga, massage, and/or muscle relaxation.
- Ask other relief workers about their experiences and feelings, doing so may help you process your own.
- Keep a journal.
- Take care of yourself. Get as much sleep as possible. Take rest breaks, eat properly, and avoid drinking large amounts of caffeine or alcohol. Physical activity, such as running, walking, or engaging in sports, is also helpful.
- If something especially upsetting happens, take a short break, do a relaxation exercise, or talk to someone about it. Do not dwell on what happened.
- If you have been working away from home, give yourself a few days to make the transition once you return. Tell your family that you need some time to yourself before you return to a normal schedule. Expect that other family members also will have been dealing with stress.
- If you experience prolonged symptoms, contact a behavioral health professional.

Preparing Your Family and Neighborhood

An important part of being prepared happens at home. If you do not know that your family is safe and secure, you may not be able to concentrate on your job or even come to work. To ease your mind, create your own emergency plan.

Be Aware

When electricity goes out, ATMs and credit card readers will not work. In that event, cash may be the only accepted form of currency.

Family Emergency Plans

The first step is to identify the situations that are most likely to occur where you live. Then find out the recommended procedures for dealing with them. Most people know about and have some experience with the natural disasters that occur in their areas—hurricanes in Florida, earthquakes in California, and so on. Know the ways to protect yourself within your home and your neighborhood.

However, other local hazards may be less obvious—a chemical plant, for example. Sources of information on local hazards include local and county emergency management agencies and health departments. Ask for information on emergency procedures in the community, including how citizens are alerted.

Emergency alerts may include warning sirens, television and radio announcements, automatic telephone dialing and cell phone texting systems, social media (e.g., Facebook, Instagram, and Twitter), the Weather Radio

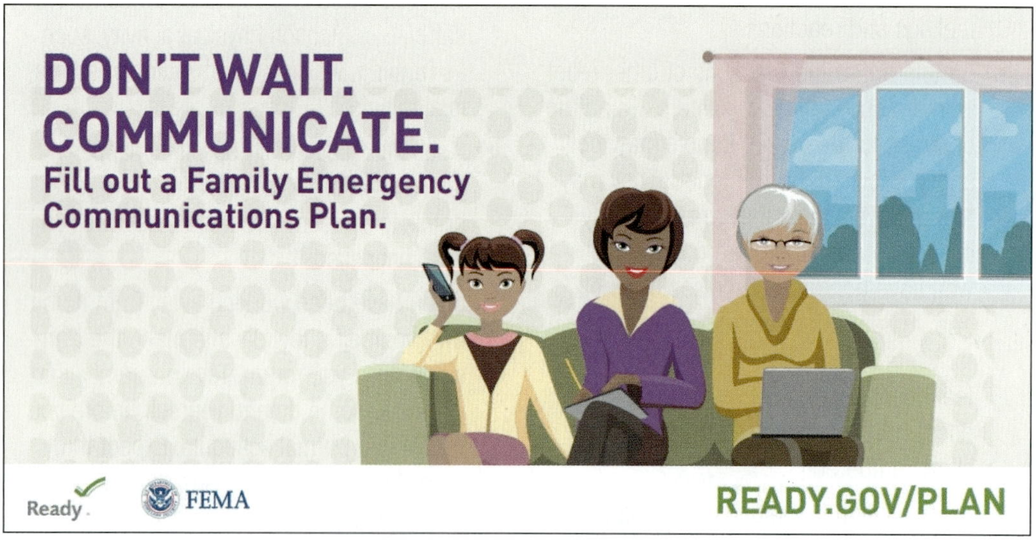
DON'T WAIT.
COMMUNICATE.
Fill out a Family Emergency Communications Plan.
Ready
FEMA
READY.GOV/PLAN

This emergency preparedness campaign from Ready.gov helps to identify the importance of family emergency communication plans.

(run by the National Oceanic and Atmospheric Administration), mobile applications on smartphones, and door-to-door notifications.

When you are familiar with the potential emergencies in your community, meet with the members of your family and create a plan together. Working as a team and sharing responsibilities will help all family members understand what they need to do. Include children in some of the planning. Tell them that incidents like fire or severe weather may occur where you live and that preparing for these events can make them safer.

Families should decide ahead of time how they will contact one another, where they will meet, and what they will do in different situations. These actions should be written into the plan. Families should designate two meeting places—one right outside the home and another outside the neighborhood, such as a library or community center. Everyone in the family must know the address and phone number of these places.

Families should ask an out-of-town friend or a relative to serve as a "communication center" if family members become separated. Every member of the family should know who that person is and have the phone number readily accessible.

As explained in Chapter 5, it is also important to have a plan for any pet or animal in your care.

Staying Safe in Your Own Home In some events, government authorities will advise people not to evacuate but to seek shelter in their homes. Emphasize to everyone in your family that they should follow the instructions. Explain that authorities make these decisions based on the type of situation. For example, during a tornado, people are safer underground

A Closer Look

Taking Cover from Falling Objects

In a sudden emergency with moving walls, objects, or debris, such as an earthquake, take immediate actions to protect yourself, such as:

- Go under a sturdy desk or table and cover your head with your hands.
- Stand in a doorway or under a stairwell.
- Move away from file cabinets or bookshelves that might fall.
- Move away from exterior walls and windows.
- Face away from windows and glass.
- Do not use elevators.

in basements. In a chemical release, an aboveground location is preferable because some chemicals are heavier than air and may seep into basements even if the windows are closed.

Train everyone in the family on how to stay safe at home. If you are in an area where earthquakes occur, have all members of the family know how to quickly protect themselves from falling items. If in a mobile home, get out of it and go to the closest building. Make sure that everyone in your family knows not to leave a place of safety until they know the danger has passed.

What to Do if You Evacuate In case you're advised to evacuate, a designated member of the family should call or email the out-of-town contact to tell this person where the family members are going. This is important because a disaster can interrupt or destroy the power, cell phones, and Internet. You need to have thought through many options in case some of

A Closer Look

Family Contact Information

The following is an example of what everyone should carry in case of an emergency:

If I am called to work to respond to an emergency, our family has made the following arrangements so that all are cared for while I am on duty.

My child(ren) will be cared for by:

____
(Name)

____
(Cell Phone Number)

____
(Address)

My parent(s) will be cared for by:

____
(Name)

____
(Cell Phone Number)

____
(Address)

My pet(s) will be cared for by:

____
(Name)

____
(Cell Phone Number)

____
(Address)

Our meetings places are:

____

We will all call ______ at ______ to report where we are and that we are safe. (Phone Number)

We will also try to leave status messages on Facebook, if possible, and at ______ to report where we are and that we are safe.

A Closer Look

Additional Ways to Prepare your Family

- Be sure that every family member knows how and when to call 911.
- Identify a friend or family member that you could stay with during an emergency in case of evacuation.
- Check your homeowner's insurance policy to see what it will cover.
- Prepare family emergency supplies, such as water, batteries, battery-powered radio, blankets, packaged food, and any needed medications.
- Take a first aid course with your family. The American Red Cross and other organizations offer courses.

them do not work. If separated during the evacuation, every member of the family should reach out to the contact so that everyone knows that the members of the family are safe.

Evacuation planning should also include special arrangements for family members who are ill or disabled and for pets. All household members should keep a copy of the family disaster plan and emergency contact information in their wallets, briefcases, or backpacks. Contact information should include names, addresses, phone numbers, and where to meet in case of an emergency. Children may have to show the information to a teacher or other trusted adult. Once everyone knows what to do in an emergency or disaster, families should practice their plans, including a mock evacuation.

Family Emergency Supplies

It is important that you and your family be prepared with food, water, and alternative power. Collect supplies and store them in a convenient location. Start small. You will need both an emergency kit in case you must leave and shelter-in-place supplies in case you need to stay in your home for a while without power, food, and water.

Emergency Evacuation Kits An **emergency kit** is a small collection of essentials that you and your family may need in the event of an evacuation. At a minimum, the kit should contain the following:

- Copies of the family's emergency plan with information about contacts and the meeting places
- An extra set of car and house keys
- Credit and ATM cards and enough cash to be able to buy gasoline for your vehicle and purchase other essentials, if possible, until after the emergency is over

An emergency kit filled with supplies including nonperishable food, a first aid kit, and emergency plans.

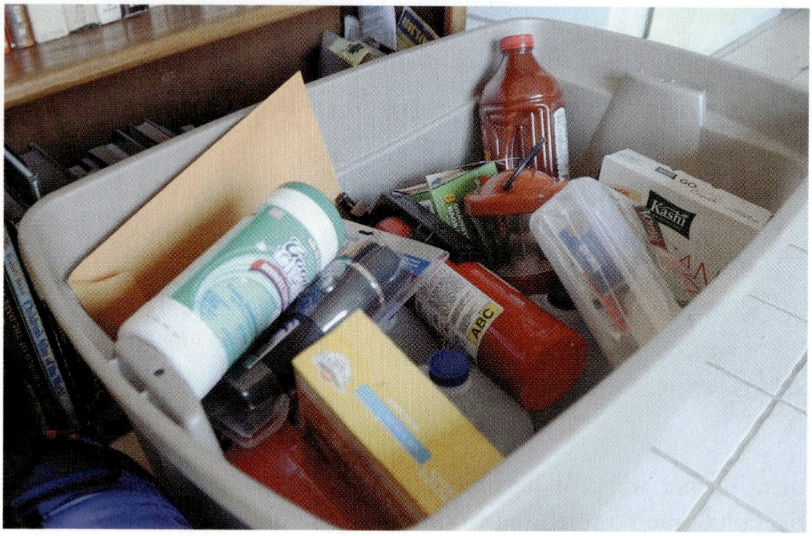

- Hand-cranked or battery-powered flashlight and AM/FM radio
- Extra batteries for the flashlight and radio
- A list of the prescription medications each member of your household takes, why they take them, and the dosages
- If you decide to keep extra medications in the emergency kit, be sure to rotate them before they expire
- First aid kit
- Childcare supplies, if needed, and other special care items

An emergency kit contains what you can quickly pick up and carry with you. You can pull together a more extensive collection of supplies to keep in your home.

Shelter-in-Place Supplies Your shelter-in-place supplies should include enough emergency supplies to take care of family members without outside help for at least three days. Everyone in the family should know that these supplies are for emergencies only. Once prepared, supplies should be updated and checked twice a year for the expiration dates of food and medications. Food and stored water should be replaced periodically to keep them fresh. A good time to schedule an update is when daylight saving time begins and ends.

The supplies to keep in your home should include everything in the home emergency kit, plus the following:

- Water: Have one gallon of water per person per day for at least three days for drinking and sanitation. You may want to store more if a family member is on medications that require water or increase thirst. Store water in plastic containers.

- Unscented chlorine bleach and a medicine dropper: When diluted (nine parts water to one part bleach), bleach can be used as a disinfectant. If necessary, you may sanitize water by using 16 drops of unscented chlorine liquid bleach per gallon. Water purification tablets or iodine tablets also work. Purchase these at stores that carry camping supplies.
- At least a three-day supply of nonperishable food: Select foods that require no refrigeration, preparation, or cooking, and need little or no water. Examples include energy, granola, or fruit bars; dried fruit; nuts; peanut butter; crackers; boxed juices; ready-to-eat foods; and foods for special dietary needs.
- Manual can opener
- Plastic sheeting and duct tape to protect an area within a larger room to keep dust, smoke, or toxins to a minimum when sheltering in place
- Moist towelettes, hand sanitizer, garbage bags, and plastic ties for personal sanitation
- Basic tools (wrench, pliers, and so on)
- Sleeping bag or warm blanket for each person
- Matches in a waterproof container
- Mess kits, paper cups and plates, plastic utensils, and paper towels
- Paper, pens, pencils, and sharpeners
- Books, games, puzzles, or other activities for children
- Personal hygiene items, including toothbrush, toothpaste, comb, brush, soap, contact lens supplies, and feminine hygiene supplies
- Extra eyeglasses, walking aids, and similar items
- Pet food and extra water for pets, if needed

Include anything else that you feel is important. Ask for suggestions when you discuss the plan with your family. Your healthcare knowledge can be a guide. The American Red Cross and other organizations have websites that can provide additional suggestions.

Reassuring Children

Although disasters may cause apprehension for adults, they often affect children more seriously. Children may become uneasy when they do not know what to expect. They may be especially upset if they must leave their home. In a disaster, children are often afraid that someone will be injured or killed, that they will be separated from their family, or that they will be left alone. To help children cope with disaster:

- Comfort and reassure them that they are safe.
- Explain the situation to children. They need to know that they are not responsible for what happened.

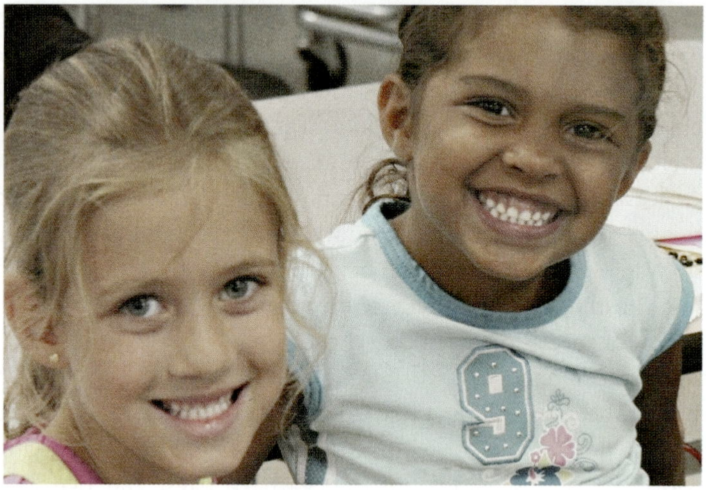

These children in Audubon Park Elementary School in Orlando attended a FEMA puppet show for children. Puppet therapy is one of the techniques for preparing children and helping them understand storms and what happens afterward.

- Explain what will happen next. For example, "Tonight, we will all stay together in the shelter."
- If possible, include the entire family in the discussion.
- Encourage children (even teens) to talk about their fears.
- Have at least one adult stay with the children (even teens) before and during a disaster.
- If possible, keep children busy with their daily routines.
- Adults should not show or tell their fears to children.

Neighborhood Planning

Schools, day-care centers, workplaces, and public buildings should all have site-specific emergency plans. People should know about the places where their family members spend time and ask about emergency plans at those places. Know what is in the plan, and be sure that it does not conflict with the procedures in your family plan.

For example, parents with children should know whether the school will keep students at the school or send them home. Parents must also know how to authorize a friend or relative to pick up the children if they cannot. They should provide the school with up-to-date contact information for themselves and at least one other neighbor, relative, or friend.

Talk to your neighbors about how you can all work together in the event of an emergency or disaster. Some neighborhood organizations, such as a home association or crime watch group, may have disaster preparedness as part of their organized activities and will share the information with you.

Neighbors can decide who will check elderly or disabled neighbors. They can share contact information and make backup plans for children in case someone cannot get home.

Chapter Summary

Government, institutions, and individuals need to be prepared for emergencies and disasters. Individuals must be prepared both on the job and at home. Healthcare workers must be familiar with the emergency plans of their employers and their role in the plans. In addition to the contributions they make to disaster efforts at work, healthcare workers can also make important contributions as volunteers.

Disaster work is stressful. Learning to recognize the signs of stress and how to cope with stress is critical for healthcare professionals both at work and as volunteers. It is possible to reduce one area of stress—concern for family. By being prepared at home and by planning for emergencies, healthcare workers can do their jobs without worrying about their families.

Additional Resources

To extend the content presented in this chapter, take advantage of the resources available through the chapter's eBook resource links and the end-of-chapter link. These resources include informational supplements and flash cards for terms and abbreviations.

Key Terms	
basic life support	emergency kit
burnout	Emergency Management Assistance Compact
crisis intervention counseling	Emergency System for the Advance Registration of Volunteer Health Professionals
defusing	Good Samaritan laws
emergency action plan	just-in-time training

Recognizing Terms

Choose the word or phrase from the list of key terms that best matches each of the following descriptions. Your instructor may ask you to submit your work for grading or may provide you with an answer key for self-assessment.

1. A type of training offered by the American Red Cross __________
2. Volunteer registration for health professionals in each state __________
3. A mutual aid agreement among states for disaster relief __________
4. Stress-reducing technique lasting from 10 to 30 minutes __________

5. Counseling where workers share their feelings and discuss how to recover from the experience of working in a disaster __________
6. Small collection of essentials for an emergency evacuation __________
7. A condition in which people experience emotional exhaustion __________
8. Legal protection when helping in emergencies __________
9. Specific last-minute training for tasks the volunteer will be performing __________
10. Identifies and explains the actions to be taken by a company in an emergency __________

Reviewing Concepts

Choose the response that best answers the question or completes the sentence. Your instructor may ask you to submit your work for grading or may provide you with an answer key for self-assessment.

1. Which of the following is not a basic medical skill?
   a. taking vital signs
   b. providing CPR
   c. drawing blood
   d. providing ventilator support

2. During a disaster response, directing victims to the appropriate area for treatment would be considered a
   a. professional skill.
   b. basic medical skill.
   c. support skill.
   d. technological skill.

3. Which federal agency requires companies to have a written emergency action plan?
   a. Occupational Safety and Health Administration
   b. Environmental Protection Agency
   c. Federal Emergency Management Agency
   d. National Disaster Medical System

4. Why is preregistration important for assisting in disaster response?
   a. It increases the likelihood that you will be paid on time.
   b. It lets family and friends know your whereabouts.
   c. It helps to ensure that you will know what you will be expected to do.
   d. It tells authorities how many volunteers will be needed.

5. Before traveling to an affected region, volunteers should
   a. make sure that their automobile insurance covers rental vehicles.
   b. get a rabies shot.
   c. create a family emergency plan.
   d. complete their income tax forms.
6. Health professionals who want to preregister to work in a disaster area should contact
   a. CISD.
   b. local or state health department.
   c. ESAR-VHP.
   d. OSHA.
7. A brief, stress-reducing technique that takes place immediately following a disturbing incident is known as
   a. defusing.
   b. critical incident stress debriefing.
   c. crisis intervention.
   d. posttraumatic counseling.
8. An emergency kit should contain
   a. iodine tablets.
   b. a manual can opener.
   c. a warm blanket.
   d. photo IDs.
9. What are some signs of burnout? Select all that apply.
   a. feel tired even when you get enough sleep
   b. work less efficiently
   c. pull away from family and friends
   d. drink or use drugs to feel better
10. When preparing for an emergency at your home, how many days of supplies should you gather?
   a. 1
   b. 3
   c. 5
   d. 6

Exploring Emergency Preparedness Issues

Complete the following activities to further explore the concepts found in this chapter. Your instructor may ask you to submit your work for grading or may provide you with guidance for self-assessment.

1. Contact your local or state department of health and find out how you can register to volunteer to help in an emergency or disaster. Summarize the necessary steps in one or two paragraphs.
2. Prepare an emergency plan for your family. Include every detail described in this chapter: care for your children and pets, where to meet, an out-of-state contact, and so on.
3. Contact your children's schools and ask for a copy of their emergency plan. Write a short summary of the plan. Then discuss if you think the plan meets the criteria discussed in this book.
4. Visit the SAHMSA website to access their free "Disaster Kit: SAMHSA's Emergency Mental Health and Traumatic Stress Services" at **http://EmDPrp2.ParadigmEducation.com/SAMHSA-DisasterKit**. This toolkit arms disaster recovery workers with materials that aid in responding effectively to the general public during and after a disaster, and in dealing with workplace stress. Then write a one-page summary of the tips that apply to your scope of practice.

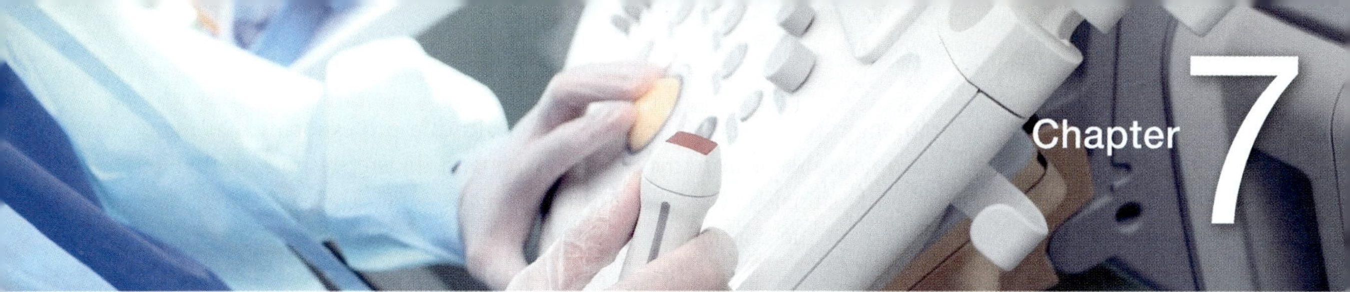

Chapter 7

The Roles of Allied Health Professionals

What You Will Learn

- How various allied health professions may contribute to emergency and disaster preparedness, including:
  - Emergency medical technicians and paramedics
  - Health information managers and technicians
  - Healthcare interpreters
  - Medical laboratory technicians
  - Medical imaging and radiation therapists and technicians
  - Phlebotomists
  - Respiratory therapists and technicians
  - Surgical technologists
  - Pharmacists and pharmacy technicians
  - Physical therapists and assistants
  - Medical assistants
  - Behavioral health counselors
  - Veterinary technicians
- What community members can do to assist in an emergency or disaster

Although doctors and nurses are the healthcare professionals that many people think of in terms of emergency and disaster response, all allied health professionals have skills and roles that are vital. Their roles may vary depending on the community and the emergency or disaster. This chapter provides an overview of allied health professions and how the members of each profession can help in times of medical surge.

Although this chapter provides an overview of how each type of professional can contribute in a community emergency or disaster, it cannot cover all aspects of every profession. Each profession requires skills that need to be honed for responding in a disaster and that require more in-depth explanation, training, and practice.

Key Acronyms	
ALS	advanced life support
NLTN	National Laboratory Training Network
RERT	Radiological Emergency Response Team

Emergency Medical Service Specialists

As described in earlier chapters, Emergency Medical Services (EMS) personnel, considered first responders, provide medical care for patients' immediate medical needs at incident sites. Once the patients are stabilized, EMS personnel transport them to hospitals via ambulances, helicopters, and planes.

Emergency Medical Technicians

Emergency medical technicians (EMTs) are trained to evaluate the condition of a patient and provide emergency and stabilizing medical care. EMTs follow protocols under the direction of emergency physicians via radio or dispatch station. EMTs administer basic life support to ensure a patient's survival before a patient arrives at the hospital. By applying cardiopulmonary resuscitation (CPR) and defibrillation, they maintain airway breathing and circulation. This may include abdominal thrusts to dislodge something causing a person to choke, known as the Heimlich maneuver. EMTs control external bleeding by putting pressure on a wound. EMTs also help prevent further injury or disability by immobilizing potential spinal injuries and bone fractures. When possible, EMTs obtain the medical histories of patients being transported to facilitate the ability of the hospital's medical staff to treat patients quickly. EMTs write up the patient care reports (PCRs), which are transmitted to the hospital's emergency department (ED).

When the EDs are experiencing a medical surge from a disaster, EMTs may be called in to assist in providing medical care. EMTs may also be asked to provide vaccinations or medications at a Point of Dispensing (POD) site if there is a major outbreak of an infectious disease.

Paramedics

Paramedics are EMTs who have additional training and responsibilities, including the provision of **advanced life support (ALS)**, which involves more complex medical procedures to save lives. Like EMTs, paramedics receive doctors' instructions and orders via radio. The medical procedures performed by paramedics include applying advanced airway management techniques, such as inserting a tube into the trachea to help someone breathe (known as intubation); performing defibrillation; using equipment to suction stomachs; interpreting tests conducted on heart monitors; starting and monitoring intravenous medications; and performing other emergency medical procedures at the site of the incident or in the ambulance on the way to the hospital. Paramedics are allowed to administer some drugs orally or by injection. Paramedics also create PCRs that will be transferred electronically or with the patient if electronic transmission is impaired.

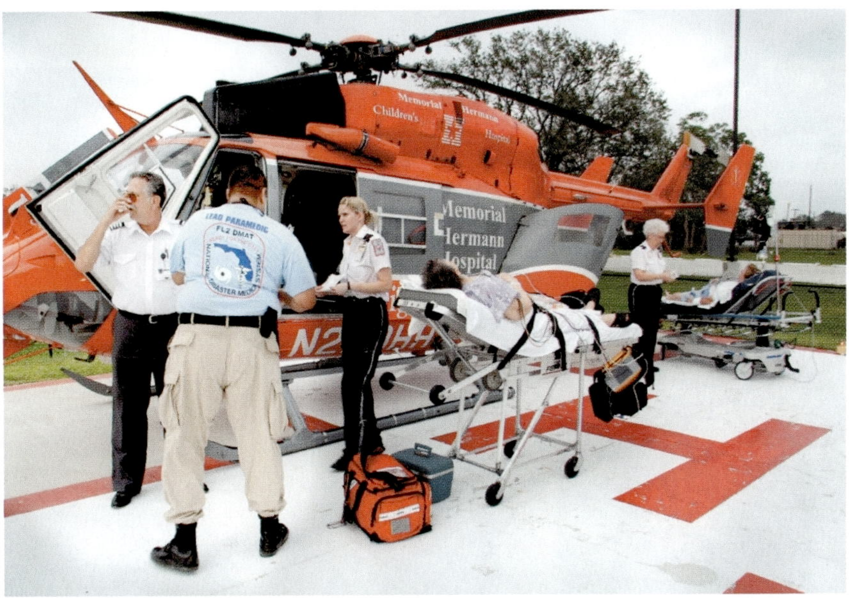

In 2005, a Medivac helicopter pilot, a flight nurse, and a paramedic work with a Florida2 DMAT unit to rescue patients in Beaumont, Texas, after Hurricane Rita.

Health Information Professionals

All medical care must be documented to maintain continuity of patient care (and protect the facility and providers from liability once the patient is discharged or transferred). Physicians, EMTs, paramedics, nurses, medical assistants, and pharmacy technicians are often the ones interviewing patients and their caretakers for health information. However, health information management (HIM) professionals are the ones who organize and save the medical records; protecting records so that they do not get lost or compromised and making the information easily available even after the crisis is over. HIM professionals also work to protect the patient's privacy.

Health Information Technicians and Managers

Health information technicians collect known information to create or maintain individual patient medical records. They will check the individual records for accuracy and completion. Health information managers and analysts can then use the collective data to process and interpret reports for various departments and hospital functions and required reporting to government agencies.

In a disaster, HIM professionals work together to find methodical, organized ways to preserve existing records and to create new ones for efficient retrieval and use. During a medical surge from a mass casualty incident, many new medical records may have to be created quickly. HIM professionals

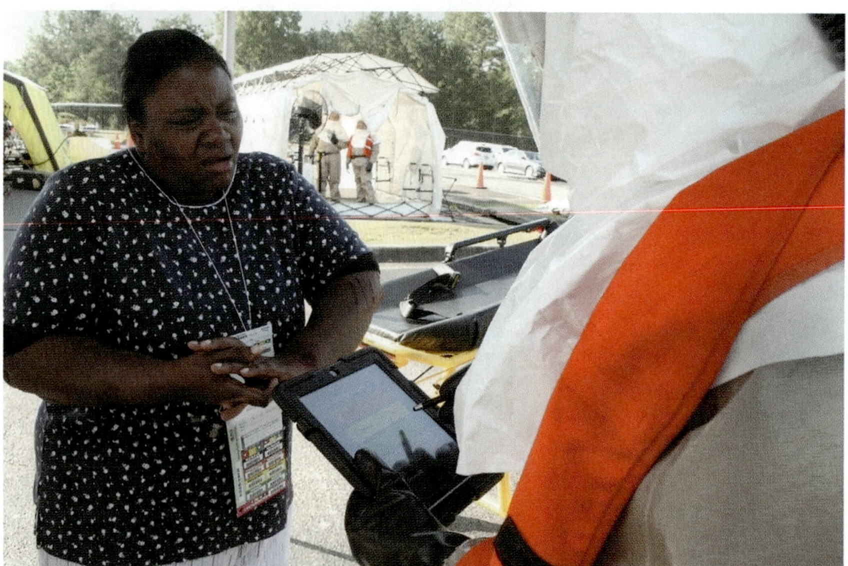

Healthcare professionals use handheld devices and patient tracking software. This innovation allows health information technicians and managers to collect information and access the healthcare facility's databases even if the general power is out or computers are damaged.

create medical record numbers for new patients to ensure that each patient has an identifier with only one medical record.

HIM professionals are critical to the transfer of patient information in a hospital or long term care facility evacuation. They can electronically forward the records needed to the receiving hospitals, or if electronic transmission systems are down, they can go up to the medical units and make copies of the medical records that can accompany patients when they are transferred to the receiving hospital. They can also print or write out a summary of the hospital stay to travel with the patient.

Additionally, HIM professionals can organize and implement the medical records process at a medication POD site, medical shelter, or other temporary health sites. HIM professionals are also needed to facilitate the completion of information for death certificates and release them electronically. They serve as the liaison between nursing at the location where the person died, pathology (if there is an autopsy), and security in the release of the body to the funeral home.

Medical Records Coders

Medical coders are the HIM professionals who enter the appropriate codes into the patient records for reimbursement from private and government insurance and for public health data tracking. Medicare requires two special codes for services and documentation affected by national disasters or emergencies. These codes are "DR" for disaster related and "CR" for catastrophe/disaster related. Coders need to know and apply the special Medicare rules when working with these specialized codes.

In daily practice, hospitals are now allowing medical records coders to code from home, which is important for staff retention. But it is also very beneficial when a disaster or other emergency damages a healthcare facility, because coders can continue their work uninterrupted, and facilities can submit their claims for reimbursement of services provided both before and during the disaster.

Healthcare Interpreters

Communicating in the native language of the individuals who have experienced a disaster is crucial. In the aftermath, victims need to understand what healthcare professionals are asking or telling them about their conditions. And they need to understand emergency alerts to take action, instructions on what to do, and how to fill out documents when applying for assistance.

Healthcare interpreters, or translators, help physicians, nurses, and other healthcare professionals communicate with patients for whom English is a second language and with patients who are deaf or hard of hearing. Healthcare interpreters facilitate communication between health professionals and victims

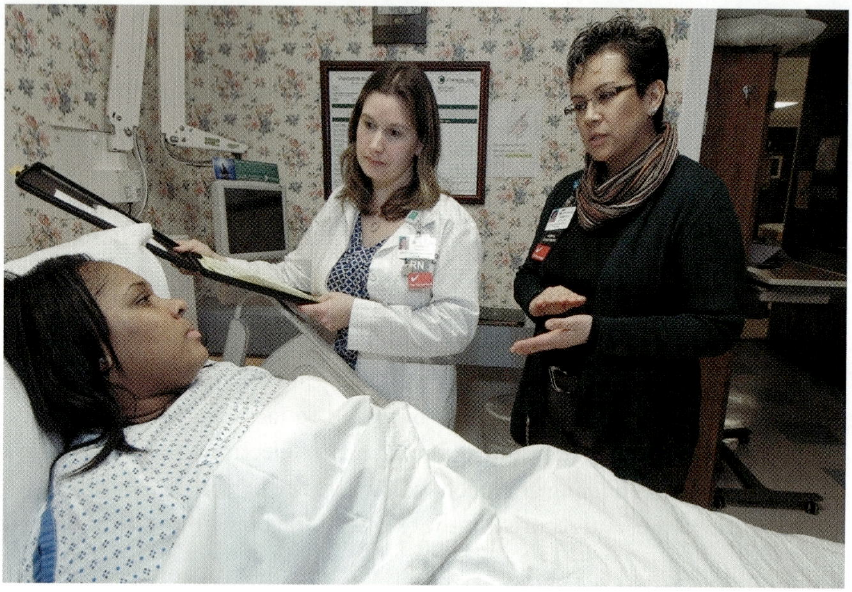

At Christiana Care Health System's Christiana Hospital in Newark, Delaware, a medical interpreter communicates in Spanish and English to facilitate communication between the patient and her nurse for ensured quality of care and understanding. Christiana Care has a dedicated Cultural Competency Manager and an extensive staff of interpreters for different languages as well as telephonic interpreting services. With these prioritized resources, Christiana Care is better poised to handle emergencies and disasters.

being interviewed about their medical and medication histories. An interpreter can convey what the person has experienced and is experiencing in the proper medical terminology. The interpreter also explains what the health professional wants the patient to know and do in ways the patient can understand. By knowing what to do, patients can avoid errors, not miss treatments, and access support services. Interpreters may also provide crucial cultural information that helps health professionals understand the patient and that facilitates a patient's willingness to follow a treatment plan.

Healthcare facilities rarely have full-time interpreters to serve patients who are deaf or hard of hearing. Some facilities have an interpreter on call or on contract for scheduled appointments. Others call freelance interpreters. Some hospitals use video remote interpreters and the patient, interpreter, and provider can see one another on video.

Medical Imaging Technicians

Health professionals in medical imaging perform diagnostic x-rays and scanning examinations that are key in diagnosing patient injuries and illnesses in an emergency or disaster. These health professionals include radiographers, radiology technicians, sonographers, and sonography technicians. Medical imaging technicians are trained in anatomy, patient positioning, examination techniques, equipment protocols, imaging safety and protection, and basic patient care. Radiographers and radiology technicians handle x-rays, magnetic resonance imaging (MRI), and computed tomography (CT) scanning. Sonographers and sonography technicians (also known as ultrasound technicians) direct high-frequency sound waves for imaging internal parts of the body. Medical imaging technicians perform their duties under the direction of the specialists (such as a radiologist).

Many types of emergencies create the need for an extraordinary number of diagnostic imaging tests to be performed swiftly and simultaneously. For example, many internal and external injuries are associated with windstorms, earthquakes, and the cleanup afterward. Explosions can cause blast injuries that must be evaluated through imaging tests, such as in the Boston Marathon case. In addition, medical imaging becomes critical if thousands of chest x-rays are required due to a widespread infectious disease, such as influenza.

During such medical surge, imaging professionals may work in their usual settings, be reassigned to the ED, or be called upon to perform duties in other locations because they have preregistered to assist as part of medical response or disaster mortuary teams.

Without positive identification, it is difficult to release the bodies of victims to their loved ones. Imaging professionals help identify bodies through body and bone scans and dental x-rays. Imaging professionals may volunteer for a Disaster Mortuary Operational Response Team (DMORT) or with the state's Emergency System for Advance Registration of Volunteer Health Professionals. In 2005, DMORT pathologists used radiography to identify badly decomposed bodies that had been in the water up to seven weeks after Hurricane Katrina.

Expand Your Knowledge

The US Department of Health and Human Services has a Radiation Emergency Medical Management (REMM) resource webpage. It provides guidance on how to develop emergency response plans at **http://EmDPrp2.ParadigmEducation.com/radiationRplan**.

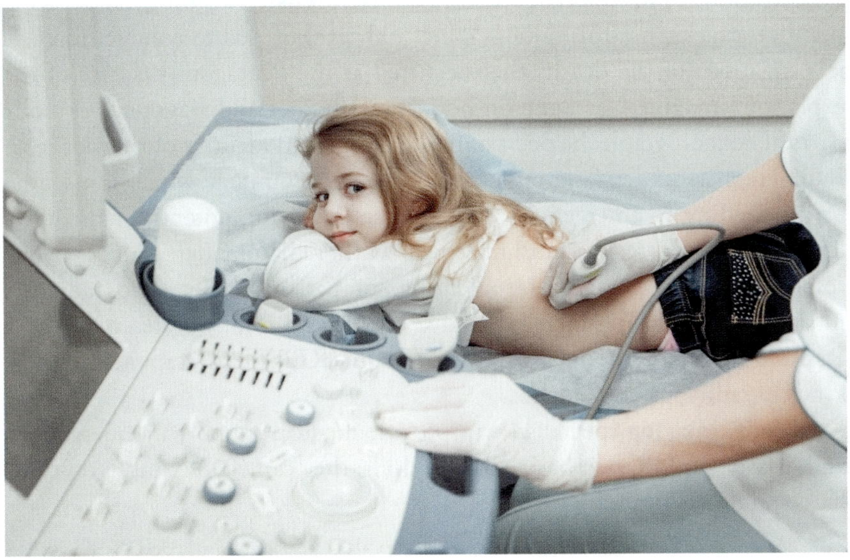

Having access to a variety of imaging specialists and equipment is essential for handling a medical surge of injured or ill patients.

Heroes Corner

Rapid Recovery for Imaging Services

In preparation for Hurricane Sandy, the New York University Langone Medical Center (NYULMC) radiology department shut down all systems and computers. This included unplugging the equipment from the wall where possible, and where this was not possible, the main electrical switch was shut off. They stored supplies needed to run the equipment in refrigerators that were sealed. They made sure that the MRI machines were completely maintained. They monitored the compressors and chillers so that if they lost power, personnel could turn off the water pumps and compressors before they overheated.

At 11 p.m. on October 29, the department leaders went home to bed thinking that all imaging equipment was safe. The next morning, however, the entire outpatient magnetic resonance facility was under 15,000,000 gallons of water. They had lost all network connectivity, Internet access, five magnetic resonance imaging machines, one computed tomography scanner, the necessary equipment to run these machines, the imaging workstations, and all of their supplies.

In the next few days, over 60 faculty and staff responded by relocating the surviving computers, ultrasound equipment, picture archiving equipment, and communication system components. They created new workspaces and a new area to perform outpatient imaging. They set up temporary rooms for radiologists to read the images. To deal with having less equipment available to scan the same number of patients, they revised the radiology staff's work schedules and extended night and weekend hours so that more patients could be seen with the staff and equipment available.

Expand Your Knowledge

The US Department of Health and Human Services has a Radiation Emergency Medical Management (REMM) resource webpage. It provides guidance on how to develop emergency response plans at http://EmDPrp2.ParadigmEducation.com/radiationRplan.

Imaging tests may also produce criminal evidence for police and FBI investigations. This specialty is known as **forensic radiology**. Following the 9/11 attacks in 2001, radiographic analysis was used to conduct forensic investigations of the deaths that occurred at the Pentagon. Because of the explosion, imaging was done on both intact bodies and fragments of body parts. The radiographs helped establish the age and identity of the victims. Radiographers understand radiation and Geiger counters, which is essential for responding to emergencies and disasters involving potential radioactive leaks. Radiology technicians may help with radiation detection. Anyone responding to such disasters or caring for patients exposed to radiation must wear special personal protective equipment. Many states organize a **Radiological Emergency Response Team (RERT)** to respond to these kinds of radiological incidents.

Finally, imaging specialists can provide medical support in emergencies and disasters. With their basic medical skills, they can check vital signs, draw blood, and perform CPR.

Medical Laboratory Managers and Technicians

Medical laboratory managers oversee both lab staff and test results and analysis to ensure that specimen testing is being completed in accordance with quality standards. Medical laboratory technicians, also known as medical technicians (med techs), conduct tests that help detect, diagnose, and treat many conditions and diseases. Most of their work is done in hospital or community labs.

During a medical surge, medical laboratories must quickly process specimens. If multiple injuries have occurred, lab personnel may have to type and cross-match hundreds or thousands of blood samples so that transfusions can be performed. If a chemical accident has occurred, a lab might be asked to analyze hundreds of samples of body fluids for chemical content. During a disaster, there may be physical problems in the laboratory, such as damaged workspaces, requiring the relocation of the lab to another space. A laboratory may also lack sufficient storage space in the refrigerators and freezers for all the samples.

Because of the medical surge and limited time available to process an increased number of tests, medical laboratory managers and technicians must quickly assess which tests they can perform given the circumstances and how fast. They need to prioritize which tests are most important to conduct first, possibly processing the tests with fewer technological aids. They also must work to preserve the integrity of the tests that were already in progress.

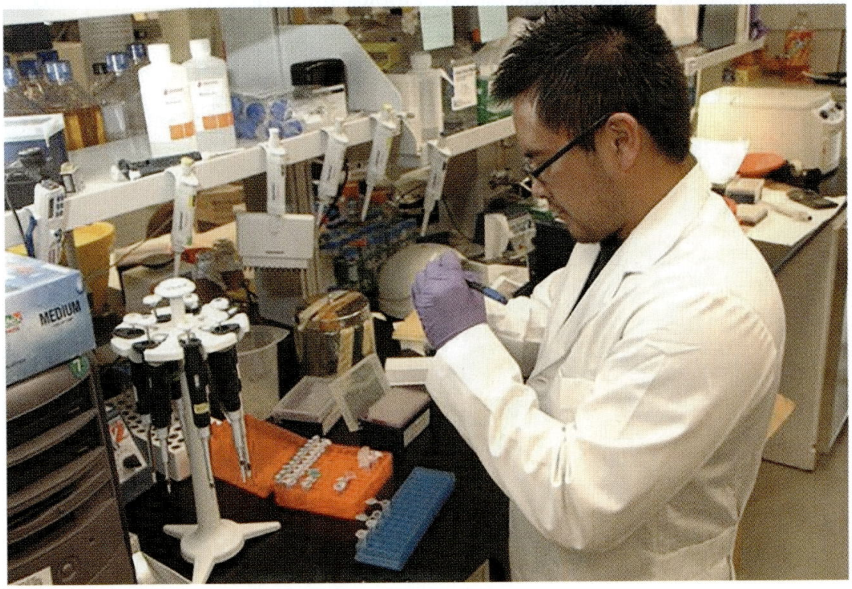

A medical laboratory technician is responsible for conducting tests to help detect, diagnose, and treat conditions and diseases.

Laboratory technicians need to know the protocols for notification and communication of results. They first report the findings to their supervisor and/or laboratory manager and the physician who ordered the tests. The physician and the hospital then work with the county and state departments of health and the Centers for Disease Control and Prevention (CDC), if there are results of concern. For emerging diseases, as explained in Chapter 3, samples may be sent to a reference laboratory for confirmation and next steps. Technicians also must safely transfer samples to and from the lab, properly store specimens and test results, and help with the proper and timely disposal of medical waste.

> **Expand Your Knowledge**
>
> For more information on free CDC laboratory training online and in person courses, visit http://EmDPrp2.ParadigmEducation.com/CDCLabTraining.

Since medical laboratory technicians assist in identifying suspicious substances, they may want to get additional training to qualify to work at a reference laboratory. One resource is the **National Laboratory Training Network (NLTN)**, which provides training courses in clinical, environmental, and public health laboratory topics.

Phlebotomists

A professional whose work is necessary for the medical lab is the phlebotomist. A phlebotomist collects the blood specimens used to process blood work. In disaster situations, having donated blood available when there are many injured patients is critical. A great number of blood samples must be tested and the skills necessary for safe blood withdrawal and preservation are essential. Phlebotomists are needed in temporary treatment sites and hospitals when many people require blood tests for transfusions. They are also necessary in the community when blood samples must be collected from many people at once, such as in an influenza outbreak in an assisted living facility.

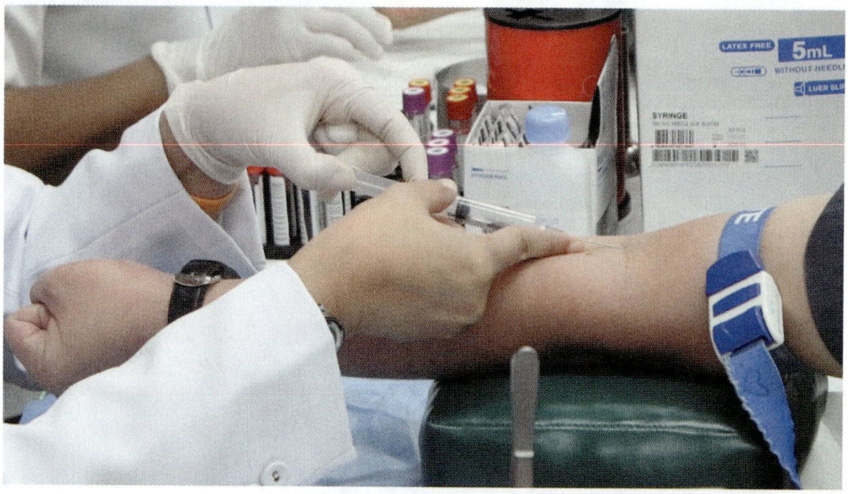

Phlebotomists provide essential medical services as part of the medical response at hospitals, clinics, and temporary treatment sites.

In an airplane crash or explosion, phlebotomists assist in the identification of victims by collecting blood samples for DNA testing on family members.

Respiratory Therapists and Technicians

Respiratory specialists are needed in many types of disasters. Respiratory care providers may be called to work as part of medical response teams in EDs, inpatient and outpatient care facilities, and medical shelters.

Respiratory Therapists

Because of their skills in airway management and ventilator support, respiratory therapists are critical in the initial efforts to resuscitate and stabilize patients in emergencies and disasters They can assess patients, recommend treatments, provide supplemental oxygen, manage ventilators and artificial airway devices, and evacuate a person on a ventilator. Additionally, they can aid physicians in assessing and treating patients throughout the entire medical response, recommending when therapy should be initiated or modified or is no longer needed.

Respiratory therapists may check patient's oxygen levels, suction fluids, and provide tracheostomy care. They can collect and interpret blood-oxygen samples and conduct a spirometry test to assess the functioning levels of a patient's lungs.

They may operate, monitor, and maintain respiratory equipment; administer medical gases, aerosols, and respiratory medications; maintain clearance of the natural and artificial airways of a patient; and provide primary assistance in CPR. Additionally, respiratory therapists should be trained to operate all types of mechanical ventilators, because they may be moved to a facility

A Closer Look

Respiratory therapists assess a patient's breathing by:

- Putting their hands on the patient to measure chest expansion
- Tapping on the chest, to evaluate the condition of the lungs
- Using a stethoscope to listen to the lungs, to determine whether the breath sounds are normal or abnormal
- Using a stethoscope to listen to voice sounds (any change in voice sounds or intensity while listening with a stethoscope may indicate pneumonia)
- Determining how difficult it is for the patient to breathe

that uses ventilators that are different from those where they regularly work. In disasters, power outages are common and breakdowns occur. A respiratory therapist, often with the technician's assistance, should be prepared to maintain ventilator support for patients, even if power fails. That means knowing whom to contact for backup power and being able "**to bag**," or manually provide ventilation for the patient, until the power returns. That work is done with a handheld **bag-valve mask** device that can be squeezed, released, and squeezed again to force oxygen into the patient's lungs.

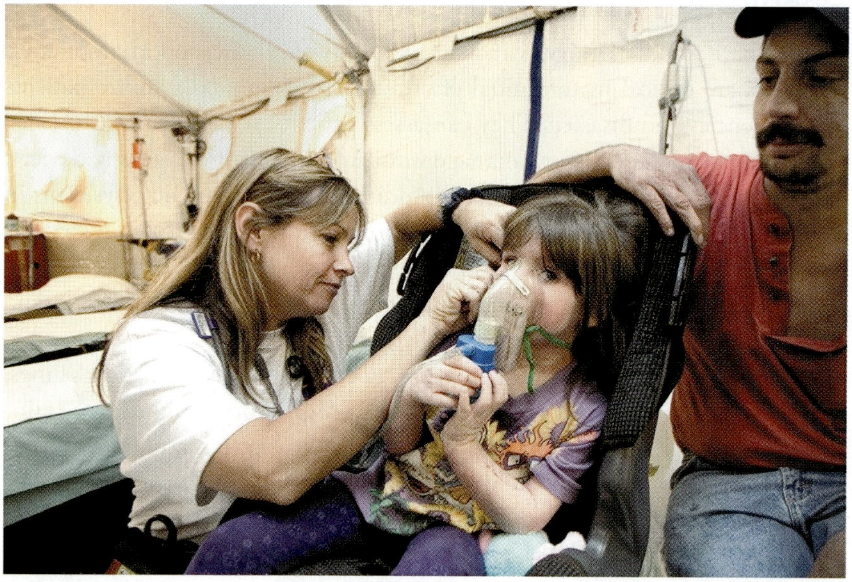

A respiratory therapist assists a young patient with her mask. This scene was inside the Disaster Medical Assistance Team tent at Punta Gorda, Florida, following Hurricane Charley in August 2004.

Respiratory Technicians

Under the supervision of a respiratory therapist, technicians assist in monitoring the applied oxygen and breathing treatments to ensure that patients are breathing properly. Technicians prepare and test equipment before beginning procedures, analyze samples, document treatments, and maintain records. In an emergency or disaster, the technician's responsibility to keep the equipment in working order becomes even more significant.

In incidents involving inhalation of toxic materials, the medical response often involves extensive resuscitation and respiratory support. There might be a rapid administration of respiratory medications by the therapist, with the assistance of the technician. In pandemic influenza, the resources of hospitals will likely be overwhelmed by a surge of patients with respiratory problems, and the respiratory staff may be asked to work longer shifts or to come in during nonscheduled hours.

Surgical Technologists

During emergencies and disasters involving mass casualties, there will likely be a surge of patients needing immediate surgery. Surgical technologists prepare operating rooms by selecting and opening sterile supplies, sterilizing surgical equipment, placing sterile drapes on the patient in preparation for surgery, and passing instruments and sponges to surgeons. After surgery, the technologists apply bandages and assist in moving the patient from the room. The technologists may be reassigned from their normal posts in surgery or orthopedic units to the ED to assist in treating patients there.

Since they are trained in CPR and other first aid skills, surgical technologists can support emergency and disaster response on medical response teams in addition to their usual roles in hospital surgical units and EDs. Surgical technologists may serve on a DMAT. As part of this effort, they receive additional training and can prepare casts and splints, help with surgical procedures in or out of the hospital, and provide wound care.

Pharmacists and Pharmacy Technicians

As explained in earlier chapters, maintaining access to prescriptions can be key to the health of many patients, and pharmacies are essential in this process. As noted in Chapter 2, pharmacies need a disaster plan. This includes providing strategies for acquiring pharmaceuticals and supplies, and guidelines for dispensing them. Personnel involved in inventory management should be fully aware of the pharmacy's plans.

Like other facilities, pharmacies should have backup generators. However, as part of preparedness, pharmacists and pharmacy technicians need to know the pharmacy's plan if a disaster interrupts or destroys the computers and online systems. These systems assist in maintaining patient profiles, online prescription transmission, checking for potential drug interactions, and inventory tracking. Technicians, however, should know how to assist in filling prescriptions and helping dispense vaccines if the electricity or computer access fails. Within hospital pharmacies, personnel will need to know how to document the filling of unit and crash carts on paper, how to remove medications from electric automated dispensing machines, and how to follow through with filing paper medication administration records from the nursing staff until the power returns. Technicians may also have to serve as delivery runners, carrying prescription orders and medication administration records along with the dispensing carts.

If there is early warning of an approaching hurricane or other weather event, technicians may be asked to contact chronically ill patients with

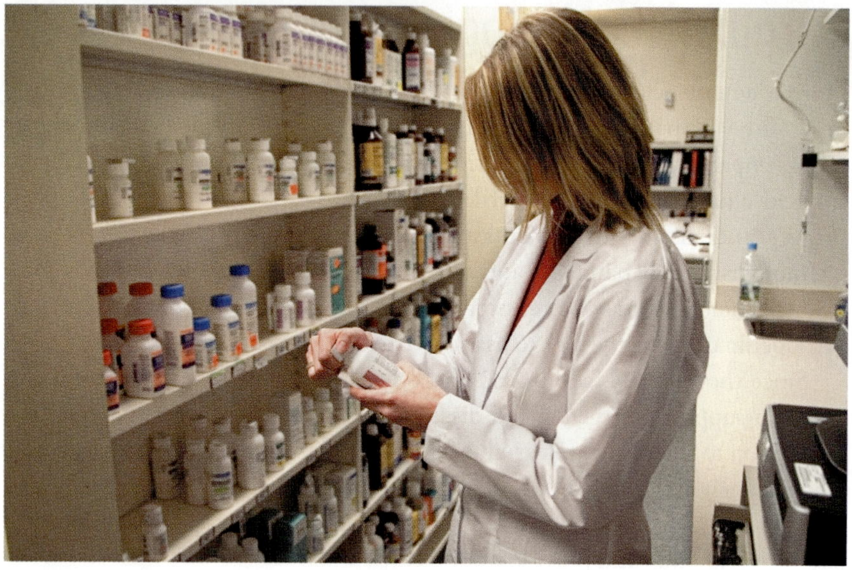

An experienced technician is responsible for ordering and stocking not only the drug product inventory, but necessary medical supplies and supplements as well.

important reminders to properly pack necessary medications, collect prescription records, and potentially refill appropriate medications early. Pharmacy technicians may also communicate with insurance providers to ensure that the cost of the prescriptions filled early will be covered by insurance.

In daily practice, records are backed up on-site or to remote physical or virtual locations. However, if there is danger of flooding and potential for damage to on-site electronic storage systems, patient profiles can be backed up electronically onto an external drive that can be transported and plugged in at another location.

During evacuations, patients may leave home without the appropriate medications and may need assistance in obtaining supplies of medications for medical conditions. The patients may not remember the names of their medications or the dosage. They may not be able to get in touch with their own pharmacy and doctors, or their medication and medical records may have been destroyed. Some people may have to replace medications that require refrigeration. Pharmacy technicians have the skills to work with patients to create a patient profile or look up records on the pharmacy database. Hospital pharmacy technicians may need to provide medication lists to be transferred with evacuating patients.

Pharmacy technicians can also assist if a disaster calls for the large, rapid administration of medications, vaccines, or anti-infectives at a POD site. They can prepare and record the vaccinations, obtain permissions from patients and guardians, provide educational materials and, in some states, check blood pressures and administer the vaccines.

Physical Therapists and Assistants

Physical therapists provide treatments for injuries to muscles, tendons, nerves, and bones to increase flexibility, movement, and function, and to decrease pain. Physical therapist assistants help by educating patients in the proper way to perform exercises, monitoring their movements in the therapist's prescribed treatments, and providing therapeutic massage.

During an evacuation, physical therapist assistants can help move patients safely and comfortably. They are familiar with the physical capabilities of patients and can advise on the types of assistance that patients and staff will need during evacuations. Physical therapist assistants can also be helpful in medical shelters assisting evacuees with activities of daily living. The massages they can provide to relieve stress for response and relief workers and patients are a great service.

Medical Assistants

If a disaster occurs, the administrative area of a medical office will be a busy place. Many patients will contact their usual clinic or medical practitioner for treatment, information, or referrals. Medical assistants perform a variety of clinical and administrative tasks in a wide range of settings. They take patient histories and vital signs, prepare patients for a variety of procedures, assist the healthcare provider with examinations and treatments, collect specimens, perform some diagnostic tests, and administer medications as directed by the healthcare provider. They also schedule and receive patients, maintain medical records, handle telephone calls, and interact with patients.

In the event of an order to evacuate, medical assistants can help patients find sources of medical equipment, such as oxygen. Medical assistants need to stay informed so that they can provide accurate information. They may advise patients with chronic diseases about what to have in their evacuation kit or shelter-in-place supplies.

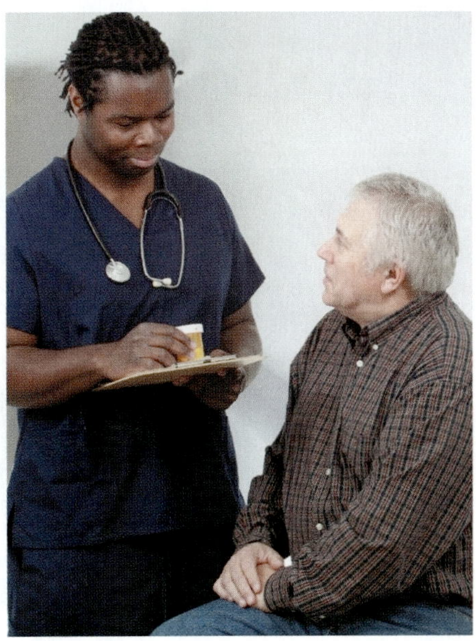

Medical assistants can perform a wide variety of roles during emergencies and disasters because of their experience in working with patients in a variety of clinical and administrative contexts.

Medical assistants can also apply their clinical and administrative skills as volunteers on medical response teams. They can perform many nonmedical support roles effectively because of their experience working with patients. In some states, medical assistants may be temporarily authorized to give injections and draw blood by the state's department of health.

Behavioral Health Counselors

Following a disaster, local behavioral health professionals organize to help victims and their families cope and begin the road to recovery. Behavioral health professionals include youth or adult counselors, drug and substance abuse counselors, members of employee assistance programs, healthcare and educational intake and admissions counselors, child protection workers, youth services workers, and rehabilitation program coordinators and assistants. They serve in healthcare and educational settings, family service and adoption agencies, and state or local government agencies.

Most counselors will not be working from an office when assisting emergency and disaster victims and their families. This behavioral health assistance is often done in nontraditional settings, such as shelters and assistance centers. Services in the immediate response and recovery phases are focused on assisting victims and response workers in meeting their basic needs,

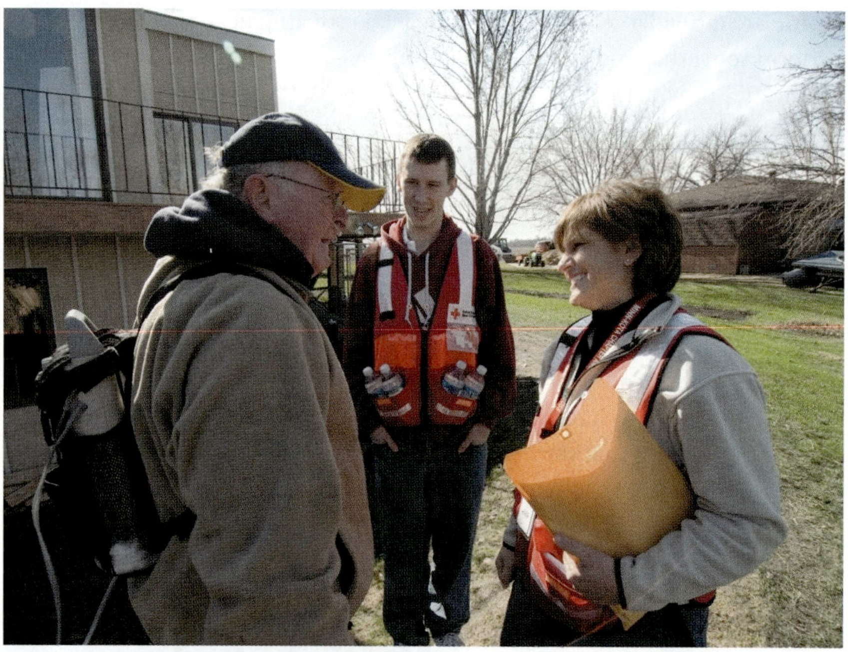

In April 2009, after the Red River flooded Clay County, counselors canvassed the neighborhoods and spoke with riverfront residents near Moorhead, Minnesota.

including helping people feel safe and secure, obtaining food and water, linking them to needed services, helping them get first aid and medications, and connecting victims to family, friends, and other social support networks. Behavioral health professionals can also provide information on resources available to victims; help connect victims to community organizations and local agencies; and develop and distribute educational materials.

Some states have organized behavioral health teams that are ready to go into the field to help victims of disasters that occur in their communities. Behavioral health professionals who have state licenses or state certifications (clinical social workers, psychologists, professional counselors, marriage and family therapists, school counselors, and school psychologists) can join these teams or form their own.

Emergencies and disasters are so stressful that they not only create difficulties, stress, grief, and sometimes emotional trauma in the short term, but they also can cause problems that may not appear until later on in life. Long after the emergency or disaster, behavioral health professionals may find themselves working with clients who experience new or worsening problems because of it. Being aware that this may happen will better equip these professionals to carry out their roles.

Veterinarians and Veterinary Technicians

During and after an evacuation, animals left on their own can develop traumatic injuries, aspiration pneumonia, and toxic and sewage-related gastroenteritis. In addition, they may experience behavioral changes that make them difficult to handle. Pigs, chickens, turkeys, and other livestock have been killed by wildfires and the flooding following hurricanes or other storms.

Protecting the public's health from vector and animal-related infectious diseases is also important during a disaster. Infectious diseases that have followed hurricanes or other flooding disasters have resulted in mosquito-borne diseases (e.g., eastern equine encephalomyelitis), leptospirosis, cryptosporidiosis, giardiasis, and hoof rot.

Veterinary technicians assist veterinarians in caring for the livestock and pets. Their duties include observing animals to identify changes in behavior; preparing animals for examinations or surgery; giving animals nursing care or first aid; collecting and testing lab samples; taking and developing x-rays; giving medications, shots, or treatments; and collecting and maintaining the medical records of the animals being cared for.

Veterinarians and veterinary technicians serve together on VMATs. These VMAT members are serving at the Louis Armstrong New Orleans International Airport in September 2005.

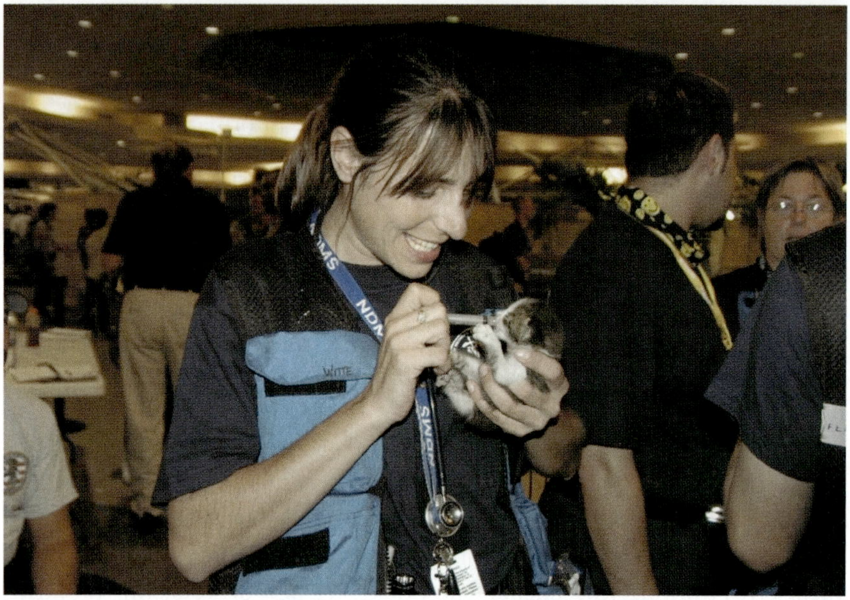

Expand Your Knowledge

If you would like to become trained for volunteering with the American Humane organization to participate as part of its disaster response, its website lists training courses you could take: **http://EmDPrp2.ParadigmEducation.com/AHTraining**.

Veterinary technicians can volunteer for Veterinary Medical Assistant Teams (VMATs) and other animal care groups. They can also volunteer with the animal rescue team of The Humane Society of the United States (HSUS). The HSUS Animal Rescue Volunteers are required to take certain FEMA courses on the Incident Command System, National Incident Management System, and other key topics.

The Role of the Community

Although the professions listed in this chapter encompass the main allied healthcare professions involved in emergency and disaster response, others are also involved (such as dental clinics that may need to provide care for their patients). In addition to allied healthcare professionals, other members of the community need to prepare and respond to emergencies and disasters. Businesses may provide supplies for free or at low cost. When usual supply chains are not available, grocery stores may supply food for volunteers or medical staff and patients. Bus companies may offer their services to transport people to safety.

The whole community must be prepared and contribute whatever services and supplies they can. You should now have a better understanding of the role your profession (or future profession) has in an emergency and disaster and how you can contribute to your community's preparedness efforts.

Chapter Summary

The skills of all allied health professionals are invaluable in emergency and disaster response. Members of each profession can make an important contribution. Because emergency response is a team effort, it is helpful to know how different professionals apply their knowledge and skills in an emergency.

Additional Resources

To extend the content presented in this chapter, take advantage of the resources available through the chapter's eBook resource links and the end-of-chapter link. These resources include informational supplements and flash cards for terms and abbreviations.

Key Terms	
advanced life support	forensic radiology
bag-valve mask	to bag

Recognizing Terms

Choose the word or phrase from the list of key terms that best matches each of the following descriptions. Your instructor may ask you to submit your work for grading or may provide you with an answer key for self-assessment.

1. A device that can be squeezed, relaxed, and squeezed again to force oxygen into the patient's lungs __________
2. Manually provide ventilation for a patient when there is no electrical power __________
3. Medical treatments that ensure a patient's survival before a patient arrives at the hospital __________
4. Use of x-rays and other imaging tests to examine human remains so that police and FBI can investigate incidents of terrorism __________

Reviewing Concepts

Choose the response that best answers the question or completes the sentence. Your instructor may ask you to submit your work for grading or may provide you with an answer key for self-assessment.

1. What is a role of physical therapist assistants during a disaster response?
   a. help evacuees with activities of daily living
   b. assist patients with breathing problems
   c. take patient histories
   d. distribute medicine and vaccines to evacuees

2. Which allied health professional conducts tests to help detect, diagnose, and treat diseases?
   a. emergency medical technician
   b. pharmacy technician
   c. laboratory technician
   d. health information technician

3. In a disaster response, which health professional helps to identify dead bodies?
   a. respiratory therapist
   b. radiation therapist
   c. physical therapist assistant
   d. surgical technologist

4. Which health professional provides wound care and prepares splints and casts?
   a. physical therapist assistant
   b. medical assistant
   c. surgical technologist
   d. medical imaging therapist

5. Which health professional has the most medical training to assist people at the scene of a disaster?
   a. laboratory technician
   b. surgical technologist
   c. medical assistant
   d. emergency medical technician

6. What skills are helpful to a medical assistant?
   a. computer repair skills
   b. mechanical ventilator skills
   c. advanced life support skills
   d. administrative and clerical skills

7. A paramedic administers which of the following?
   a. POD
   b. CT
   c. CPR
   d. ALS

8. What role can a health information technician play during an emergency?
   a. help victims obtain a supply of medications
   b. keep patient records from being destroyed
   c. schedule and receive patients at a shelter
   d. take x-rays to determine injuries

9. What should be part of the emergency preparedness activities of a pharmacy technician?
   a. making backup copies of customers' medication records
   b. conducting routine maintenance of the electric medical devices of customers
   c. supplying insurance information for the LEMA
   d. helping customers preregister for a medical shelter

10. What is the role of health care interpreters during an emergency?
    a. help interview victims so physicians can learn about the patient's medical history
    b. help the medical team avoid errors in understanding and/or communication about needed healthcare services
    c. provide cultural information, which helps health professionals understand the patient and which facilitates a patient's willingness to follow a treatment plan
    d. All of these.

11. Who performs diagnostic imaging exams?
    a. surgical technologists
    b. phlebotomists
    c. radiology technicians
    d. medical assistants

12. Behavioral health counselors perform which services following a disaster?
    a. help finding resources for basic needs
    b. provide psychological first aid
    c. provide information about where to go for help
    d. All of these.

13. Whose work is necessary for the medical laboratory to process blood work?
    a. surgical technologists
    b. phlebotomists
    c. radiology technicians
    d. medical assistants

14. What is a key task of veterinarian technicians following a disaster?
    a. locating lost pets
    b. tracing identification on pet collars
    c. observing animals to identify changes in behavior
    d. bringing pets back and forth from shelters

15. Which skilled professional is critical in initial efforts to resuscitate victims?
    a. surgical technologist
    b. radiation therapist
    c. respiratory therapist
    d. physical therapist

Exploring Emergency Preparedness Issues

Complete the following activities to further explore the concepts found in this chapter. Your instructor may ask you to submit your work for grading or may provide you with guidance for self-assessment.

1. Contact your state or national professional association. Find out about the activities that they have planned for your profession in the event of a disaster and discuss this information in several paragraphs.
2. Which of your healthcare colleagues are you likely to work with during a disaster? What similar tasks will each of you work on together? Which different tasks will each of you work on? Summarize your response in one page.

Glossary

access and functional need an individual's inability to get to services or limitations on functioning that require additional response assistance before, during, and/or after an incident

advanced life support (ALS) emergency medical procedures that exceed basic life support techniques; require an additional level of training beyond what an EMT receives; can be performed by a paramedic

all-hazards planning a general preparation and training approach that addresses many risks, which can be applied to a wide range of emergency and disaster scenarios.

ambulatory related to walking; when a patient is able to walk without assistance

antidote a substance that can counteract a form of disease or poison

assay a type of test, typically performed in a laboratory, to analyze the composition of a substance

assets personnel, equipment, and other supplies available to a community in a disaster response

assistance center a place for victims to go to access resources and get aid after a disaster

Assistant Secretary for Preparedness and Response (ASPR) government office that helps state and local agencies and healthcare systems prepare for and respond to the medical needs of an affected community or area; also known as Office of the ASPR, part of the Department of Health and Human Services

at-risk populations a term used to describe patients who are particularly vulnerable for negative outcomes before and after a disaster

autoclaving a method of treating infectious medical waste by exposing it to high heat steam and pressure to destroy microorganisms; also called "steam sterilization". See also *medical waste.*

bag-valve mask a handheld device that can be squeezed, released, and squeezed to force oxygen into the lungs of a patient with breathing difficulties

basic life support (BLS) a set of noninvasive methods for lifesaving that include emergency cardiovascular care (ECC)

behavioral health providers professionals who promote well-being by helping individuals with trauma and stress recovery; preventing and intervening in mental illness and substance abuse and addiction; also known as mental health specialists or providers

biosafety protocols safety procedures for handling infectious biological materials

bioterrorism the deliberate release of dangerous and/or highly infectious viruses, bacteria, or toxic agents that can cause illness or death in people, animals, or plants. See also *terrorism.*

Biothreat Team the laboratory team tasked with handling and testing specimens that might pose a biological threat

blast injury the physical damage sustained from an explosion's pressure, being thrown back against something, flying debris, or from fire that develops

burnout a condition of extreme emotional exhaustion; symptoms include fatigue, irritability, difficulty concentrating or sleeping, lack of enthusiasm or desire, and physical symptoms, such as headaches and gastrointestinal upsets

casualty collection point a place to gather injured victims to sort them by injury category and to stabilize their medical conditions before sending them on to hospitals for care

cardiopulmonary resuscitation (CPR) a step-by-step process used to restart the beating of a heart and breathing when both have ceased; includes chest compressions and providing breaths

Centers for Disease Control and Prevention (CDC) the federal agency responsible for tracking infectious diseases and working with states and other nations to prevent their spread and providing guidance to departments of health on emergency and disaster preparedness

Center for Domestic Preparedness (CDP) a FEMA-run center to provide training programs to the nation's response managers and providers

chemical, biological, radioactive, nuclear, and high-yield explosive events (CBRNE) emergencies and disasters that involve chemical, biological, radioactive, nuclear, and high-yield explosives and require high levels of decontamination and protective gear for responders; also shortened to CBRN without explosive events

cohorted patients patients with similar symptoms who are suspected of having the same disease and grouped together for care

cold zone an area adjacent to the warm zone that is far enough away from a release site and decontamination processes to be contamination-free; where decontaminated patients are sorted for transport to the proper treatment facility

Community Emergency Response Team (CERT) local volunteers trained with organizing and response skills, such as fire safety, light search and rescue, basic medical aid for victims

comprehensive emergency management a planning and action approach to managing disasters that encompasses four phases: prevention and mitigation, preparedness, response, and recovery.

computed tomography (CT) a type of x-ray scanning that creates a series of images of a specific area of the body; also known as CAT scans (computerized axial tomography scans)

contact tracing the tracking down and monitoring of each person who had contact with someone ill with or exposed to an infectious disease

contaminated patient someone who has been exposed to a harmful chemical, biological, radiological, or nuclear substance and may have the substance on their clothes and/or in or on their bodies

continuity of care ongoing, coordinated medical care received from the same group of healthcare professionals

credential proof of specific professional education and skills

crisis intervention counseling discussion in individual and/or group sessions that helps responders relieve stress and recover from their experience

decontamination the removal or neutralization of harmful chemical, biological, radiological, or nuclear substances or agents

defusing a brief, informal procedure (10-30 minutes) used by behavioral health professionals to help disaster workers express their thoughts and feelings about events

Department of Defense (DOD) the federal department that oversees military planning and branches of services

Department of Health (DOH) a city, county, or state department that addresses public health

Department of Health and Human Services (HHS) the federal department that addresses public health; handles or oversees the health-related aspects of emergency and disaster preparedness and response; includes the CDC and the Office of the ASPR

Department of Homeland Security (DHS) the federal agency in charge of domestic security and promoting comprehensive emergency management; includes the Federal Emergency Management Agency

disaster an emergency that requires outside assistance from the federal government. See also *natural disaster*.

Disaster Medical Assistance Team (DMAT) state or regional healthcare teams with varied healthcare professionals and paraprofessionals; deployed by the National Disaster Medical System to supplement local medical resources

Disaster Mortuary Operations Response Team (DMORT) a team that provides victim identification and mortuary services; deployed by the National Disaster Medical System

Disaster Technical Assistance Center (DTAC) a website by the Substance Abuse and Mental Health Services Administration that provides resources for the behavioral health of the community and responders

domestic terrorism a terrorist attack accomplished by a US citizen or group

don and doff the proper process of putting on and taking off personal protective equipment

droplet precautions the protective procedures health professionals follow when they are examining a patient with symptoms of a respiratory infection; includes wearing a face mask

Ebola Virus Disease (EVD) a rare, deadly, and highly infectious disease

emergency from a public health perspective, an incident that threatens public safety, health, and welfare, where a group(s) of people require immediate or a higher level of care

emergency action plan (facility) a written plan that identifies and explains the actions to be taken in an emergency; required by OSHA for companies with more than 10 employees

emergency and disaster preparedness the act of making plans to prevent, respond to, and recover from emergencies and disasters

emergency cardiovascular care (ECC) a higher level of resuscitation than CPR that requires additional training; includes clearing of obstructions, applying defibrillator or respiratory mask

emergency exercises simulated drills designed to identify the strengths and weaknesses of an emergency operations plan

emergency information form (EIF) a form that lists medical conditions, medications, and other needed information for vulnerable populations

emergency kit a collection of essentials that an individual and/or family may need in the event of an evacuation

Emergency Management Assistance Compact (EMAC) a mutual aid agreement that facilitates sharing resources, personnel, and equipment across state lines during disasters

Emergency Management Institute (EMI) a training organization run by FEMA to strengthen emergency management core competencies

emergency medical technician (EMT) a health professional who is trained in ambulance medical operations and procedures

Emergency Medical Services (EMS) the community-oriented system for providing emergency treatment and transportation to hospitals directed by a dispatcher through phone calls, usually to 9-1-1

emergency operations center (EOC) a place where leaders of the response gather to coordinate efforts, receive reports, and issue public communications

emergency operations plan (EOP) a plan that designates who will be in charge and who will coordinate the efforts of all responding parties

Emergency Preparedness Rule a set of requirements from the Centers for Medicare and Medicaid Services that healthcare facilities must adhere to if they want federal reimbursement

Emergency Prescription Assistance Program (EPAP) a federal program that provides 30-day supplies of prescribed medications and supplies to victims in a disaster

Emergency System for Advance Registration of Volunteer Health Professionals (ESAR-VHP) a system where credentialed health professionals can volunteer to work during public health and other emergencies

Emergency Use Authorization a special approval issued by the FDA to allow the use of unapproved medical products in an emergency when there are no available alternatives

emerging infectious disease an infectious disease that was previously unknown in a particular place or appears in a changed and more dangerous form

epidemic when an infectious disease outbreak spreads to a wider region

epidemiologist a disease detective, who tracks disease causing agents, investigating how they originated and how to stop them

evacuation the organized, phased, and supervised withdrawal of people from a dangerous or potentially dangerous area

external quality assurance review an evaluation of the processes and facility (e.g., a laboratory) by an official assessor from outside the organization

Federal Emergency Management Agency (FEMA) a federal agency responsible for addressing disasters, working with state and local leaders to coordinate the deployment of federal resources, providing management and response staff in the provision of shelter, food, water, and needed supplies to victims; part of the Department of Homeland Security

first responders the initial response professionals to arrive at an incident scene, such as emergency medical technicians (EMTs), paramedics, firefighters, and police

fit-tested the act of fitting and testing a respirator to ensure that the proper size, make, model, and style has been selected. See also *respirator.*

flash flooding sudden, fast-moving water

focused assessment with sonography for trauma (FAST) ultrasound scans to quickly diagnose the nature and degree of traumatic injuries

Food and Drug Administration (FDA) an agency responsible for protecting the public's food, medication, and cosmetic supply; part of the Department of Health and Human Services

forensic radiology imaging tests and analysis done to seek evidence for a criminal investigation

Good Samaritan Law legal protection for those who help someone who has been injured or is at risk for further injury

healthcare coalition (HCC) a group of healthcare facilities and organizations that have collaborative partnerships to support each other and share resources in an emergency or disaster

Hospital Incident Command System (HICS) a chain of command system in a hospital based on the ICS that clarifies roles and responsibilities in the handling of an emergency. See also *Incident Command System.*

hot zone the area immediately next to the site of a hazardous agent release; this area requires the highest level of personal protective equipment

incident an emergency event or a disaster event needing response from a specific set of responders or facility; a scalable term

incident commander an individual tasked with leading a specific response effort, including communicating with responders, assigning tasks, and designating location of incident command center. See also *Incident Command System, incident command center.*

incident command center (ICC) the location where responders meet to discuss the response and identify next steps

incident command system (ICS) a chain-of-command structure based on the National Incident Management System for organizing and coordinating emergency or disaster response at any level

incineration a method of waste disposal where waste is burned at temperatures ranging from 1,800°F to 2,000°F (982°C to 1,093°C). See also *medical waste.*

index patient the first medically identified patient in an area with a particular condition, often an infectious disease

infection control procedures standard operating procedures used by healthcare facilities to manage infectious diseases

isolation the separation of people known to have an infectious disease from those who are healthy

job action sheets the written responsibilities of healthcare professionals participating in an Incident Command System. See also *Incident Command System.*

The Joint Commission the national organization for certifying hospitals, long-term care facilities, behavioral health facilities, and ambulatory care clinics; also known as The Joint Commission on Accreditation of Health Organizations

just-in-time training the specific, last-minute training provided to volunteers to perform specific tasks for an incident response

Laboratory Response Network (LRN) a network of state and local public health, federal, and military laboratories that responds to any infectious disease, bioterrorist, or chemical threats. See also *national laboratory, reference laboratory*, and *sentinel laboratory.*

litter bearers people who move victims on stretchers

Local Emergency Management Agency / Authority (LEMA) the community governmental agency or council responsible for planning and overseeing comprehensive emergency management for a community or area

mass care services the providing of food, water, and shelter for victims, overseen by FEMA or the LEMA but run by nonprofit NGOs, particularly the American Red Cross

mass casualty incident an event that results in numerous fatalities and/or serious injuries

mass prophylaxis the large-scale dispensing of vaccines, medicines, or antidotes during public health emergencies to reduce the spread of disease. See also *Point of Dispensing.*

medical countermeasures (MCMs) medical products (drugs or devices) that can be used in a mass dispensing in case of a public health epidemic, disaster, or CBRN attack

Medical Reserve Corps (MRC) a federal program that organizes and deploys healthcare volunteers; MCRs are organized by local communities and states to enhance emergency and public health resources

medical shelter an evacuation shelter outfitted with medical staff and equipment to care for people with medical needs that cannot be properly addressed in general evacuation shelters

medical surge a sudden increase in the number of patients due to an emergency or disaster; also known as a "patient surge"

medical waste any infectious or potentially infectious materials created in healthcare settings. See also *autoclaving, incineration, sharps waste, and steam sterilization.*

memorandum of understanding (MOU) an agreement among medical facilities to receive patients from one another in case of an emergency or disaster; can also be written to conduct lab tests or share medical personnel

mitigation strategies and structures to prevent or reduce the damage of identified hazards See also *comprehensive emergency management.*

mutual aid the agreements between neighboring communities or institutions to assist one another in an emergency or disaster

National Animal Care & Control Association (NACA) a professional organization for animal shelters and animal welfare workers that keeps a database of volunteers willing to assist in animal rescue, care, and sheltering in a disaster

National Disaster Animal Response and Recovery Teams (NDARRTs) volunteer response groups created to help victims reunite with their lost pets following a disaster

National Disaster Medical System (NDMS) a federal system of rapid deployment of medical teams, equipment, and supplies to a disaster area; also moves ill and injured patients from the disaster to a safe area, and provides care for patients in hospitals away from the disaster site

National Incident Management System (NIMS) an operational structure and template for communities to organize themselves and coordinate their response activities in a similar manner; enables all levels of government, private sector, and nongovernmental organizations to work together in response

national laboratory the highest level of lab in the Laboratory Response Network; the national laboratory is responsible for isolating and identifying specific strains of biological and chemical agents. See also *Laboratory Response Network, reference laboratory, and sentinel laboratory.*

National Laboratory Training Network (NLTN) a federal resource that provides laboratory training courses in clinical, environmental, and public health laboratory topics.

National Oceanic and Atmospheric Administration (NOAA) the federal agency that tracks weather systems and alerts communities when a potentially dangerous weather event may occur; includes the National Weather Service

National Response Framework (NRF) the structure, template, and principles for how the federal government organizes itself and plans for disasters; provides guidelines for other levels of government and responding organizations to do the same

National Veterinary Response Team (NVRT) the NDMS team responsible for helping animals in a disaster

natural disaster a disaster caused by a meteorological or geological event, such as a blizzard, earthquake, flood, heat wave, hurricane, wildfire, and tornado

Nongovernmental organization (NGO) an organization that is not managed by the government

Occupational Safety and Health Administration (OSHA) the federal agency that oversees workplace safety and health regulations and guidance

Office of Emergency Management another name for the state, county, or city Local Emergency Management Agency/Authority

outbreak describes when a highly infectious disease causes people to get sick and/or die in one community or area

pandemic describes when a highly infectious disease rapidly spreads around the world, causing widespread illness and death

personal protective equipment (PPE) the clothing and equipment that protects the wearer from exposure to a hazard, such as gloves, gowns, and face masks

Point of Dispensing (POD) a temporary station for dispensing vaccines, medicines, or antidotes on a large scale, set up by a local government agency and supported by federal resources; not to be confused with Point of Distribution (also POD). See also *mass prophylaxis.*

Point of Distribution (POD) a temporary station for distributing needed supplies for disaster victims, such as water, food, blankets, diapers, and other necessities; not to be confused with *Point of Dispensing* (also POD)

preparedness a phase in comprehensive emergency management that determines how a community or an organization will respond to an emergency; includes organizing personnel, equipment, and supplies; training; conducting drills; developing communications and warning systems; creating evacuation plans; stockpiling supplies; forming alliances for mutual assistance; also a general term meaning getting ready. See also *comprehensive emergency management.*

Presidential Disaster Declaration when the governor of a state requests that the president designates a federal disaster to enable the deployment of federal resources

presumptive result a positive test result indicating a suspicious biological or chemical agent; this result requires confirmation by the next higher laboratory level

Prevention and Mitigation of Risks the first phase of comprehensive emergency management that includes a process to identify specific hazard risks (THIRA) and then implement strategies and build structures to prevent or reduce the damage from these hazards

Psychological First Aid a behavioral health intervention that involves listening and providing support and practical help for individuals who have experienced an emergency or disaster

push pack a ready-to-deploy container with enough medical supplies and medications to treat thousands of patients. See also *Strategic National Stockpile.*

quarantine the separation of people who have been exposed to an infectious disease and may be infected but are not yet ill from healthy people. See also *isolation.*

Radiological Emergency Response Team (RERT) a group of imaging specialists that train and serve during response to radiological or nuclear emergencies and disasters

reagent the specific reacting agent needed for a specialized laboratory test

Recovery the phase in comprehensive emergency management that includes activities and programs to help a community rebuild, restore, heal, and create a new normal; also general term for rebuilding and restoring. See also *comprehensive emergency management.*

reference laboratory the second level of the Laboratory Response Network, which has the reagents and technology to conduct sophisticated tests for biological and chemical agents. See also

Laboratory Response Network, national laboratory, and *sentinel laboratory.*

respirator an apparatus that cleans the air for breathing, commonly used with face masks as part of personal protective equipment

response the immediate actions to save lives, protect property, and the environment, and meet basic human needs; a phase in comprehensive emergency management when plans, responders, and resources are put into action. See also *comprehensive emergency management.*

reunification the process of bringing back together those who have been separated, especially important for recovery during an emergency or disaster

risk communication the relaying of information about a health crisis or disaster to the public in a timely and accurate way that does not unduly heighten concern and fear

scalable the ability to adjust to fit something; especially important to adjust the planning strategies, resources, and size of the response from small to large according to the size and nature of the incident

scope of practice the professional range of expertise and legally-approved responsibilities and skills for each professional

select agent an biological or chemical substance that has been identified as having the potential to pose a severe threat to public health and safety

sentinel laboratory the initial and lowest laboratory level in the Laboratory Response Network; the laboratories in the hospital, clinic, or private labs where most laboratory technicians work and where most medical testing is conducted and a suspicious agent is first tested. See also *Laboratory Response Network, national laboratory*, reference *laboratory.*

service animal any animal that is individually trained to perform tasks for the benefit of an individual with a disability, including a physical, sensory, psychiatric, intellectual, or emotional disability; often a service dog

severe acute respiratory syndrome (SARS) a potentially fatal pneumonia caused by a virus

sharps anything with a sharp, cutting edge or point; must be collected as dangerous and potentially infectious; includes hypodermic needles, syringes or tubing, scalpels, and pipettes. See also *medical waste.*

shelf life the length of time a medication is usable before it reaches its expiration date

shelter-in-place to remain in a home, facility, or designated protective area during a disaster

Simple Triage and Rapid Treatment (START) a method of triage that makes it possible for only a few rescuers to rapidly evaluate a large number of patients and move them to treatment centers for more detailed assessment. See also *triage.*

social distancing the establishment of a barrier or space between infected individuals and others to reduce the transmission of highly infectious diseases. See also *isolation, quarantine.*

staging area an area in which patients are gathered and wait to be transported during an evacuation or other emergency

standard precautions health and safety protocols that protect the patient, healthcare worker, and others from infection; including hand washing, personal protective equipment, and instrument sterilization

Strategic National Stockpile (SNS) a storage system of medicines, vaccines, antidotes, and medical supplies maintained by the federal government; deployed for disasters

Substance Abuse and Mental Health Services Administration (SAMHSA) an agency within the Department of Health and Human Services dedicated to supporting behavioral health with resources

Threat and Hazard Identification and Risk Assessment (THIRA) a set of survey processes to pinpoint risks, their likelihood of occurring in a community or facility, the potential damage, and the resources needed to address them

to bag to manually provide ventilation for a patient by squeezing and releasing a hand-held bag-valve mask to force oxygen into a patient's lungs

Trauma and Critical Care Team (TCCT) the operative and critical care team of professionals sent out by the NDMS in disasters to provide trauma care

triage a procedure for sorting victims according to their condition, treatment needs, and the resources that are available

triple packaging three-levels of secure packaging used in transporting highly infectious diseases

tsunami powerful waves that travel long distances and up onto shore, also known as a "tidal wave"

US Geological Survey (USGS) the federal agency that helps monitor and alert communities about potential geological disasters

Unidentified Patient Naming Convention a naming procedure that gives identifers to patients whose legal identities are unknown

unified command an approach in which all agencies or leaders with responsibility for handling the incident work together to establish and implement a single, coordinated response plan. See also *Incident Command System*.

universal precautions the procedures established by the Centers for Disease Control and Prevention (CDC) for working with patients where there is any possibility of exposure to blood or bodily fluids; considered standard practice of infection control; includes protective clothing and gear; handwashing after exposure, and procedures for handling sharps. See also *standard precautions*.

Veterinary Medical Assistance Teams (VMATs) volunteer response teams for emergencies and disasters organized through the American Veterinary Medical Association

Voluntary Organizations Active in Disaster (VOAD) a coalition of nonprofit groups that accept volunteers to train and deploy when needed

victim a person who is affected—including being evacuated or injured, losing loved one's or property, or becoming ill—as a result of an emergency or disaster

warm zone an area at least 300 feet away, uphill, and upwind from the site of a release site or a hazardous substance that is set up for the decontamination of patients

whole community preparedness the planning, training, and response efforts of an entire community to ensure that all citizens are prepared for emergencies and disasters

Index

D

J

K

L

M

N

O

P

Q

R

S

Photo Credits

Preface

p. xi, © michelmond/Shutterstock

Chapter 1

p. 1, © ollo/iStock; p. 2, Courtesy of FEMA News Photo; p. 4, Courtesy of Win Henderson/FEMA; p. 5, Courtesy of FEMA News Photo; p. 7, © MISHELLA/Shutterstock; p. 8, Courtesy of Elissa Jun/FEMA; p. 10, © akiyoko/Shutterstock; p. 11, © lpedan/Shutterstock; p. 12, Courtesy of Christopher Mardorf/FEMA; p. 13, © Mike Focus/Shutterstock; p. 14 (main), Courtesy of Kelly Hudson/FEMA; p. 14 (inset), Courtesy of Kelly Hudson/FEMA; p. 15, Courtesy of NOAA News Photo/FEMA; p. 16, © LawrenceSawyer/iStock; p. 17, Petty Officer 2nd Class Justin Stumberg; p. 19, Courtesy of Amanda Bicknell/FEMA; p. 21, Courtesy National Archives and Records Administration; p. 23, Courtesy of Shannon Arledge/FEMA

Chapter 2

p. 31, © Ben Carlson/Shutterstock; p. 32, © All Stock Photos/Shutterstock; p. 34, © kubkoo/iStock; p. 35, Courtesy of Jana Baldwin/FEMA; p. 36, Courtesy of Andrea Booher/FEMA News; p. 37 (main), Courtesy of Bill Koplitz/FEMA; p. 37 (inset), Courtesy of FEMA Graphic; p. 40, Courtesy of Jeannie Mooney/FEMA; p. 42, Courtesy of Shannon Arledge/FEMA; p. 43, Courtesy of Steve Zumwalt/FEMA; p. 44, Courtesy of Steve Zumwalt/FEMA; p. 46, Courtesy of Greg Henshall/FEMA; p. 47, Courtesy of Andrea Booher/FEMA; p. 48, Courtesy of Jocelyn Augustino/FEMA; p. 49, Courtesy of Shannon Arledge/FEMA; p. 50, Courtesy of Islamic Relief/FEMA; p. 51, Courtesy of Christopher Mardorf/FEMA

Chapter 3

p. 59, © Spotmatik Ltd/Shutterstock; p. 61, Courtesy of FEMA News; p. 63, © Monkey Business Images/Shutterstock; p. 65, Courtesy of Jocelyn Augustino/FEMA; p. 66, Courtesy of K.C. Wilsey/FEMA; p. 69, Courtesy of Lauren Hobart/FEMA; p. 72, Courtesy of Shannon Arledge/FEMA; p. 74 (main), CMSGT Jason M. Burger, USAF; p. 74 (inset), Courtesy of Jocelyn Augustino/FEMA; p. 76, Courtesy of Jocelyn Augustino/FEMA; p. 78, Courtesy of Liz Roll/FEMA; p. 81, Courtesy of Samuel Carr McKay/FEMA; p. 83, Courtesy of Robert Rose/FEMA; p. 84, Dr. John Herman/Massachusetts General Hospital; p. 85, Dr. John Herman/Massachusetts General Hospital; p. 88, CDC Graphic; p. 91, Aaron Sussell, Ph.D. M.P.H /CDC/CDC Connects

Chapter 4

p. 99, © PPNJ Productions/Getty; p. 102, Courtesy of Andrea Boohe/FEMA; p. 103, Courtesy of Win Henderson/FEMA; p. 105, © Tyler Olson/Shutterstock; p. 106, Courtesy of Benjamin Crossley/FEMA; p. 107, Courtesy of Andrea Booher/FEMA; p. 109, Courtesy of Win Henderson/FEMA; p. 113, Courtesy of Shannon Arledge/FEMA; p. 115, Sue Partridge, CDC-Ft. Collins;

p. 119, © lunewind/Shutterstock; p. 122, Courtesy of Jocelyn Augustino/FEMA; p. 124, Putnam County Online; p. 125, CDC/KamStrategic National Stockpile Logistics Teamelya Hinson; p. 128, Courtesy of Lillie Long/FEMA

Chapter 5

p. 135, © RapidEye/Getty; p.137, Courtesy of K.C. Wilsey/FEMA; p. 138 (main), Courtesy of Ed Edahl/FEMA; p. 138 (inset), Courtesy of Andrea Booher/FEMA; p. 139, Courtesy of Ed Edahl/FEMA; p. 141, Courtesy of Jocelyn Augustino/FEMA; p. 143, Courtesy of Barry Bahler/FEMA; p. 144, Courtesy of Ed Edahl/FEMA; p. 145, PRNewsFoto/Eli Lilly and Company; p. 148, Courtesy of John Ficara/FEMA; p. 151, Courtesy of Jana Baldwin/FEMA

Chapter 6

p. 157, © Microgen/Shutterstock; p. 158, Courtesy of Jocelyn Augustino/FEMA; p. 160, Courtesy of Mark Wolfe/FEMA; p. 161, Courtesy of Sharon Karr/FEMA; p. 163 (main), Courtesy of Hans Pennink/FEMA; p. 163 (inset), Courtesy of Ralph Simcox/FEMA; p. 166, Ilyssa Plume/FEMA; p. 168, Courtesy of Liz Roll/FEMA; p. 171, Courtesy of Liz Roll/FEMA; p. 172, Courtesy of HOPE Animal Assisted Crisis Response/FEMA; p. 174, Courtesy of Jana Baldwin/FEMA; p. 178, Courtesy of Zachary Kittrie/FEMA; p. 180, Courtesy of Ed Edhal/FEMA

Chapter 7

p. 185, © sfam_photo/Shuttstock; p. 187, Courtesy of Ed Edahl/FEMA; p. 188, Courtesy of Shannon Arledge/FEMA; p. 190, Courtesy of Christiana Care Health System; p. 191, © Romaset/Shutterstock; p. 193, © National Institutes of Health; p. 194, © SUCHAN.NI/Shuttertock; p. 196, Courtesy of Andrea Booher/FEMA; p. 198, © sjlocke/iStock; p. 199, © Val Lawless/Shutterstock; p. 200, Courtesy of Mike Moore/FEMA; p. 202, Courtesy of Liz Roll/FEMA